SECRETS TO A FLATTER STOMACH

SECRETS TO A FLATTER STOMACH

JAMIE FLYNN

Copyright 2010 Jamie Flynn

ISBN 978-1-4452-6184-3

This book is dedicated to you.

For you are the ones who inspired me to accomplish this.

I thank you for listening, acknowledging and giving me the tremendous feedback for which gave me the confidence to complete this book.

I hope this book gives you great inspiration which in turn will motivate you to achieve your goals whether large or small.

This information in this book is intended to provide general information only and is not meant to replace the medical advice given to you by your doctor/physician or health care professional. The author or employees will not be liable for any damages or claims.

We recommend you consult your doctor before deciding to change your nutrition plan, beginning any new exercise regime or participating in any detoxification program. The author has done all he can to check the accuracy of the information that appears within this book and cannot be held responsible for any changes that may occur after this print.

PREFACE

Anzac day 1998, approximately 10.30pm. After enjoying a fun but tiring day at a local football match, I was driving back to my parents' home on a narrow country road when I swerved to miss a fox directly in my path." Within seconds I had lost control and rolled the medium sized company vehicle 3 times finally landing back on all fours. "Miraculously, I walked away with just a few cuts and bruises. When the tow truck brought my car home the next day, my mother and I stood in the driveway—shocked— that I had survived with nothing more than a bruised ego." I'm not an overly religious person nor show too many emotions but I truly believe for some reason I had been given a second chance.

For the past 12 years I have committed myself to helping and educating others in respect to their health and fitness. I promised myself from that day on I would live life and do the things that made me happy. I soon left my electronics job to travel and reflect on what I wanted in life.

When I returned, I had decided that I would study part time to become a Personal Trainer and follow the path that I loved the most; sports and fitness. "I sold my car (not the wrecked one, a new one) and other valuables to start my own franchise." I still remember my father telling me I was crazy leaving a career in electronics and that I would never make anything from it. I believed I had more passion and interest for health and fitness and could fulfill my days better than electronics ever could. I decided to ignore his advice and go for it.

With an estimated 30,000 one on one personal training sessions, countless outdoor groups and hundreds of health and fitness seminars under my belt I have never looked back. I have also witnessed more than 50 health and fitness seminars questing for the right quality answers and ones not pushing towards someone else's financial goals. Today I run a successful health and fitness consultancy business called 'Three Health Australia' and lecture for one of the most recognized health and fitness training providers in Australia, 'The Australian Institute of Fitness'. I also still conduct personal training sessions, boot camps and take the odd fitness class. My personal passion lies with strength training, mountain biking, snowboarding and anything to do with sports. I was also extremely fortunate to spend some quality time overseas studying under the guidance of a very successful sports nutritionist and herbal doctor.

I was inspired to write this book for a number of reasons. The main reason stemmed from my most popular seminar called 'Secrets to a Flatter Stomach.' Many people would come up to me after the seminar wanting more information."I decided to write this book based from the success of it. I also decided to write it, not as a means for financial gain but to help educate and dispel the lack of quality information found in many other materials. I wanted to create a book that had all the information in one.

Secrets to a flatter stomach has all the information you need to help create a healthy lean body full of energy. I hope you will find the information in this book educating, motivating and helpful towards inspiring you to achieve. This book will help you understand how to not only achieve fantastic results but most importantly help you maintain it. You have my guarantee that the information in this book is scientific and achievable. As like any good investment, sometimes it does take time to adjust and understand. There is no quick fix but with significant self discipline and self motivation you will make change. To anyone reading this book, I wish you the best and hope you enjoy my book as much as I enjoyed writing it.

CONTENTS

Part One - Exercise 1

   Let's get moving – why exercise? 3

   To lift or not to lift - Strength training 5

   Telling the Truth – Myth busting 9

   Time to Rest and Recover 15

   Which exercises will reward me the most? 17

   The danger zone - How to avoid injuries 25

   Advanced Simplicity 29

   Cardiovascular Exercise 33

   Flexibility 35

Part Two - Nutrition 37

   40:30:30 – Get in the zone 39

   Insulin and Glucagon 41

   Carbohydrates 43

   Protein 47

   Fat 51

   Water 55

   Basal Metabolic Rate 57

   The dangers of yo – yo and extreme dieting 59

   The easy hand method 61

   Specific nutrition planning for ideal recovery 63

   What to Eat? 65

Part Three - Detoxification 71

   Toxins 73

   Anti-oxidants and Free Radicals 79

The importance of Circulation 83
What about Cholesterol? 85

Conclusion – It's up to you 87
Summary 91
References and Acknowledgements 95

INTRODUCTION

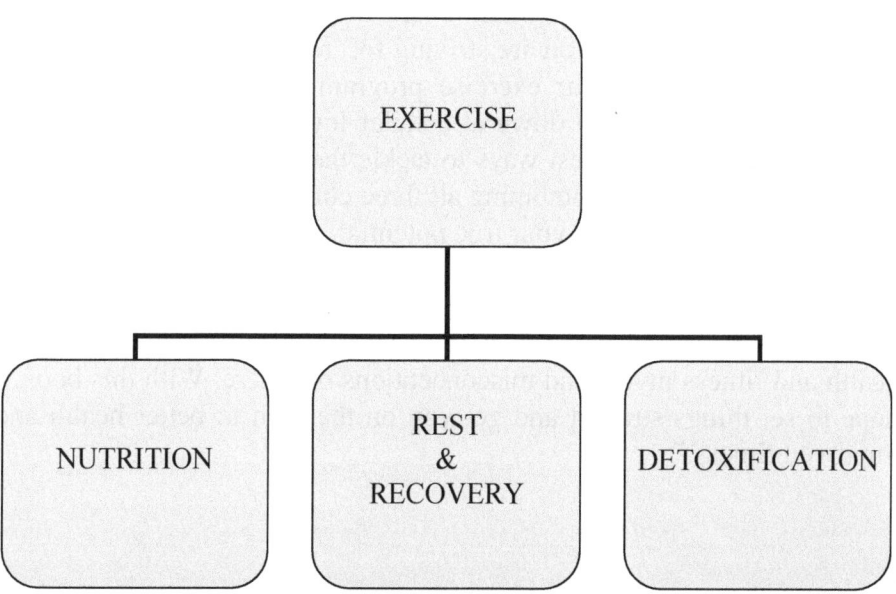

Most people are aware of the benefits that regular exercise brings to any weight-management program. Exercise can improve your overall body composition, affecting both your body weight and your shape. By 'exercise,' I mean more than just cardiovascular training such as aerobics, walking, jogging, cycling, swimming, and cross-country skiing. Optimally, your exercise program should include strength training, focusing particularly on compound movements that mimic day-to-day movements and also focusing on core stability and flexibility. The combination of cardiovascular and strength training can increase the lean mass of your body, not necessarily just the muscle size, and can help maintain correct posture, decrease poor mobility, and address problem areas. As most of you know, however, overall success is more than just exercising.

Sound nutrition based upon scientific fact is second to none. There are many 'diets' available, claiming to produce fantastic results, yet the majority not based upon current or relevant scientific research. In addition, they are rarely adapted to the individuals daily needs, however, that is not to say they do not work in one way or another but many dieters end up continually looking for the next easy fix, leaving the body composition and hormonal system worse for wear.

Detoxifying your body is also extremely important. Methods include everything from juicing, fasting, and super-food supplements to invasive treatments. Unfortunately detoxification has a bad reputation, most likely caused by poor administration, lack of knowledge and the severe extremity of the program. There may be times when you just aren't getting the results you are striving for, regardless of the effort and time that is put into your exercise program and nutrition plan. The answer may well be deep down at cellular level. It has been suggested recently that one of the best ways to tackle the problem head on is with detoxification. For this, combining all three components together may be the missing link to finding your true potential.

I hope this book will not only educate you but also motivate and inspire you to achieve your fitness goals. After being in the heart of the health and fitness industry for over 12 years, I know there are a lot of health and fitness myths and misconceptions out there. With this book, I hope to set things straight and get you on the path to better health and improved fitness."

Part One

Exercise

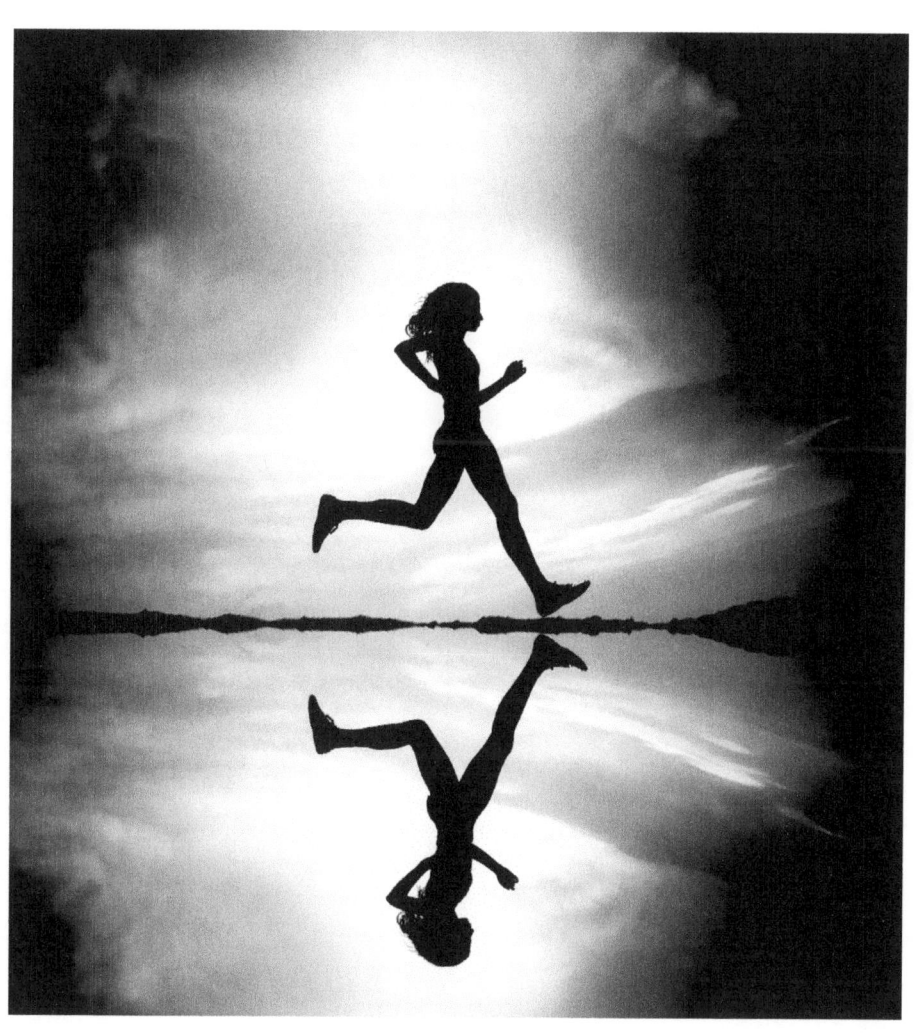

Chapter One

LET'S GET MOVING

The Benefits of Exercise

Interesting fact: Studies taken on the 15th September 2009 by the Zurich Heart Foundation Heart Health Index and the Australian Heart Association states 'approximately 54% of Australians are classed either overweight or obese, the second highest in the world.' Dr Lyn Roberts, CEO – Australia Heart Association states 'Of great concern to the Heart Association is the findings that obesity is somewhat 'normalising'. So many people who are overweight or obese do not see themselves this way. There is a misconception about what really is a healthy weight.' She continues to say 'While the stark reality is heart disease remains the major killer of all Australians.'

The fact is, we're out of shape as a society, and not nearly as healthy as many would have you believe. The birth of television, an increased sedentary lifestyle, advancements in technology, increased chemical contact, lack of exercise, fast cheap foods and other changes in the way we live have combined to produce a society with a real health and fitness crisis?

These benefits exercise can bring include strengthening joints, bones, muscles, the cardiovascular system, increasing athletic performance, increasing fat loss or helping you maintain your current body weight and composition. Regular exercise also helps boosts the immune system, helps prevent such abnormalities as heart disease, cardiovascular disease, Type 2 diabetes and obesity. It also improves mental health, confidence and can help delay and prevent depression. Exercise can also help with reducing toxic accumulation by increasing circulation, helping excrete toxins via sweat and generally helping the normal detoxification pathways. Some people also use exercise as a means for social interaction. Exercise also reduces levels of cortisol, (cortisol is a stress hormone) thereby benefiting health.

Chapter Two

TO LIFT OR NOT TO LIFT

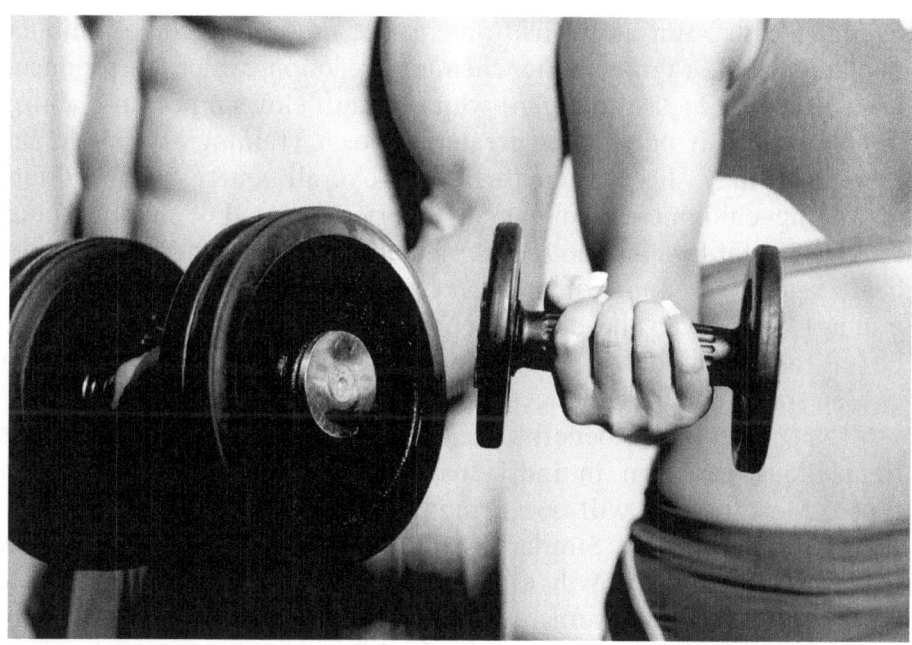

Strength Training

In my opinion, everyone should be strength training! "Strength training can be thought of as lifting, pulling, or moving a selected object or weight and can be achieved via machine, free-weights, kettlebells, bands, or even your own body weight."

Strength training appears to have a fat-burning effect that can persist for approximately 4 hours and may last up to 24 hours after the training program has long finished. This helps to burn extra calories. Unfortunately cardiovascular benefits as aerobic exercises done alone does not help increased fat burning once exercising has finished and has been shown that fat burning may slow or stabilise within 45-60 minutes after training has been completed. Combining strength training with any type of cardiovascular exercise has been proven to be the most effect combination. Completing strength training before cardiovascular training will effectively achieve a higher energy used from fat storage.

There is some conflicting evidence as to whether high intensity, vigorous exercise are more or less beneficial than moderate exercise. Wikipedia states 'that high intensity, vigorous strength training executed by healthy people can positively influence a higher hormone production (i.e. increases in testosterone and growth hormone) which is the key hormones to getting increased muscle gains and better overall health.' But as intensity increases, muscles become inhibited by lactic acid, (a metabolic chemical reaction which is produced usually from a lack of oxygen) which in turn slows a person's ability to continue their pursuit for greater fat loss. Training at a moderate, therefore, may help increase your overall energy expenditure increasing enjoyment and overall calories burnt. For an individual looking for fat loss and not concerned about performance, a moderate heart rate level approximately no more than 140bpm (beats per minute) has proven the best. I believe high intensity training should be left for people looking purely to increase their performance in their chosen sport or self challenges.

Not everyone benefits equally from exercise. There is tremendous variation in individual responses to different training types. Most people will see a moderate increase in overall fitness from aerobic exercise. Similarly, only a minority of people will show significant muscle growth after prolonged strength training, while most experience improvements in overall strength and wellbeing.

If your number one goal is fat loss, you must exercise in a 'carbohydrate depleted' state (this is when you have limited glycogen (glucose) available in your liver and muscles). To ensure you are in this state, you can perform 30–45 minutes of cardiovascular exercise before breakfast, but be sure to eat something within 30–45 minutes afterward (See my nutrition planner in Part two) or simply conduct strength training before cardiovascular training.

If your number one goal is muscle gain, you must make sure you consume enough overall calories. Eat a medium GI carbohydrate meal (e.g. banana and whole-wheat sandwich) approximately 45-60 minutes before strength training begins and drink a high GI carbohydrate, protein meal within 30-45 minutes post exercise (e.g. organic rice milk and whey protein isolate). See my nutrition planner in Part two.

For continued progress, also make sure you exercise consistently, changing your program every 4-6 weeks. Changing your routine and staying motivated will keep you on the right path to gaining muscle, losing fat, and increasing your metabolism.

Chapter 3

TELLING THE TRUTH - MYTH BUSTING

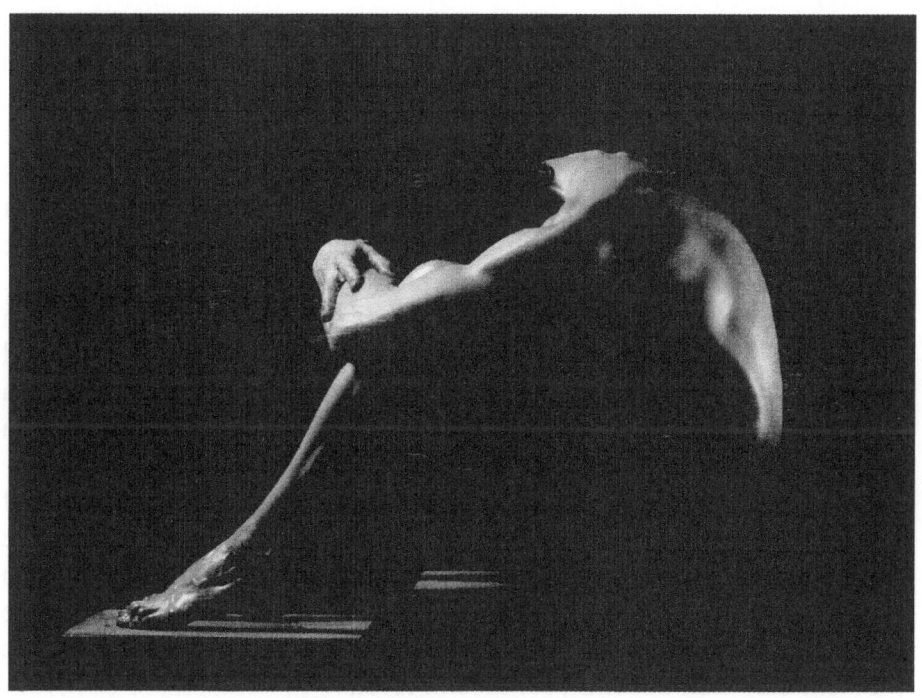

"Many myths surround exercise, some common myths include."

Exercise can cause death - Yes, it's possible to experience a heart attack or stroke if you over do it. Always check with your doctor before embarking on any new exercise program.

That strength training stops normal bone growth - One highly debate is that heavy weight training in adolescents can damage bones. This is never been proven, the most likely issue with adolescents and younger people is the general safety, postural control and lack of co-ordination and decreased concentration levels. Children should be closely monitored and educated on safe lifting speeds and selected loads.

Exercising a certain area of the body (such as the belly) will lead to loss of fat in that area - For example, doing 200 sit-ups each morning will reduce belly fat. One cannot reduce fat from one area of the body. Most of the energy derived from fat gets to the muscle through the bloodstream and reduces stored fat in the entire body. Sit-ups may improve the size and shape of abdominal muscles but will not specifically target belly fat for loss. Such practice is a total waste of time and has been shown to cause more problems that initially hoped for. Recent research by Maurice Edward Shils has proven that hormones can play a role in where body fat is predominately stored. All of us will already have a good idea of what our problem areas are and an experienced practitioner can often make an accurate visual determination of the problem.

Let's say that you discovered that there is an excessive amount of fat on your hips. This may indicate that there is a problem with the estrogen levels (a hormone predominates in females). If the problem area is the triceps, (back of the arms) the issue may well be with the androgen levels. If the problem area is the shoulder blades or hips, the problem may well be with your insulin levels.

Controlling the blood sugar levels of the body with more frequent meals, reduced daily carbohydrate and low GI food choices is critical. For lowering abdominal fat, the key is reducing cortisol levels by restricting the consumption of caffeine, sugar and detoxifying the body predominately using high alkaline foods. For the legs and gluteus (buttocks), it's important to detoxify by following a particular Detoxification program and consuming a variety of dark green vegetables such as broccoli. Many of these dietary recommendations overlap, none of them involve any method harmful to the body, and in fact, all of them will improve the overall quality of life. Taking a multivitamin/mineral tablet usually doesn't cause any harm, but it's doubtful that any one product will have the precise quantities of nutrients needed to correct a specific problem, especially with those fat-storage problems involving hormonal imbalances.

That training first thing in the morning is "catabolic" or "detrimental" and will cause a loss in muscle tissue - For the common fitness enthusiast whose body fat levels are medium to high, this is the prime time to train for body fat loss. It really depends on one's body fat level if muscle will be lost or not. For those worried about muscle breakdown, an individual weighing 75kgs @ 15% body fat or who has 10 kgs of fat carries almost 80,000 calories worth of stored fat in their adipose tissue.

This is enough stored energy to **walk** approximately 1280 km's without exhausting fat stores. The 'kreb cycle' (the complex chemical breakdown for the body to produce energy for periods of exercise longer than 2 minutes) states that energy is derived firstly from glucose in the blood, followed by stored glycogen in the liver and muscle cells, followed by energy from fat and then protein. For someone to lose valuable muscle tissue they would need to have extremely low body fat levels to begin with.

Therefore anyone with extremely low body fat levels should always eat before training commences and anyone with medium to high body fat should not. They should keep training sessions shorter, no longer than 60 minutes and limit extremely high intensity style training.

Muscle tissue will turn into fat if a person stops exercising - Fat tissue and muscle tissue are fundamentally different. The composition of a body part can change toward less muscle and more fat. This is not muscle "turning into fat". Another important issue to remember is that most people tend to continue with the normal portion sizes in their diet because of continued appetite, and will not significantly reduce portion sizes in order to compensate for the lack of exercise and calories expended.

Women who strength train or lift heavy weights will get big muscles - Women do not have the levels of testosterone and human growth hormone required to increase lean muscle tissue dramatically. Strength training will help re-shape your body. More importantly it will help increase or help maintain lean muscle tissue which can significantly increase the rate at which your body burns fat. It will also increase basal metabolic resting rate. Each kilogram of muscle you build burns approximately 80 calories per day when you are resting. The average woman loses 2.2 kilograms of muscle every decade of life, and has reduced her muscle mass by one third by the age of 50. Because muscle loss typically doubles during menopause years, a 60 year old woman may have less than half her original muscle mass, meaning slower metabolic rate and more body fat. The statistics are not much better for men, 7% less muscle and a 3 – 5% slower metabolic rate per decade. And these levels are not even considering the damage done when an individual has dieted or restricted calories, causing a huge loss in lean muscle due to lack of calories.

Men and women need different strength training exercise programs - Muscle physiology (the makeup of muscle tissue) and functional anatomy (human movement) are exactly the same for both genders which means we can and should be doing the same strength movements. Hormones and goal set are the only differences.

You can train different parts of a muscle - In the fitness industry we have a term called the 'all or none theory'. This means that the small bundles of muscle fibers, known as motor units, will either be recruited or not (the amount of motor units recruited depends purely by the amount of weight and central nervous system co-ordination). These motor units cannot be specifically targeted which is why in general we used different exercises to make sure all motor units are specifically targeted. For example, creating a peak in the bicep muscle is god's gift and genetics plays the sole role in how your biceps take shape.

Isolated exercises are best for 'toning' a muscle - There is no such thing as toning a muscle. Your muscles are already toned and controlled by the central nervous system. You simply need to decrease body fat levels, reduce fluid and reduce hormonal stresses to see your beautiful firm muscles. Compound exercises should make up at least 80% of your exercise selection.

You should not strength train if you have abnormalities like arthritis or diabetes - Strength training can initially cause some inflammation and so I recommend taking fish oils or flaxseed oil to help control inflammation. Over time you should and will notice less pain and improved function. For females with inflammation issues consume 8-12 grams of cold pressed flaxseed oil and for men 12-15 grams per day.

Muscles can remember - The term 'muscle memory' is just a term used like toning a muscle. Muscles cannot remember. Muscle memory is simply a neurological adaption. It can be explained by an individual's ability to recruit and 'squeeze' his or her muscles more easily than that of an untrained individual. This in turn causes a faster response back from training. The faster you learn to use your brain and focus on the muscle you are trying to target the faster the results you will get.

Chapter Four

TIME TO REST AND RECOVER

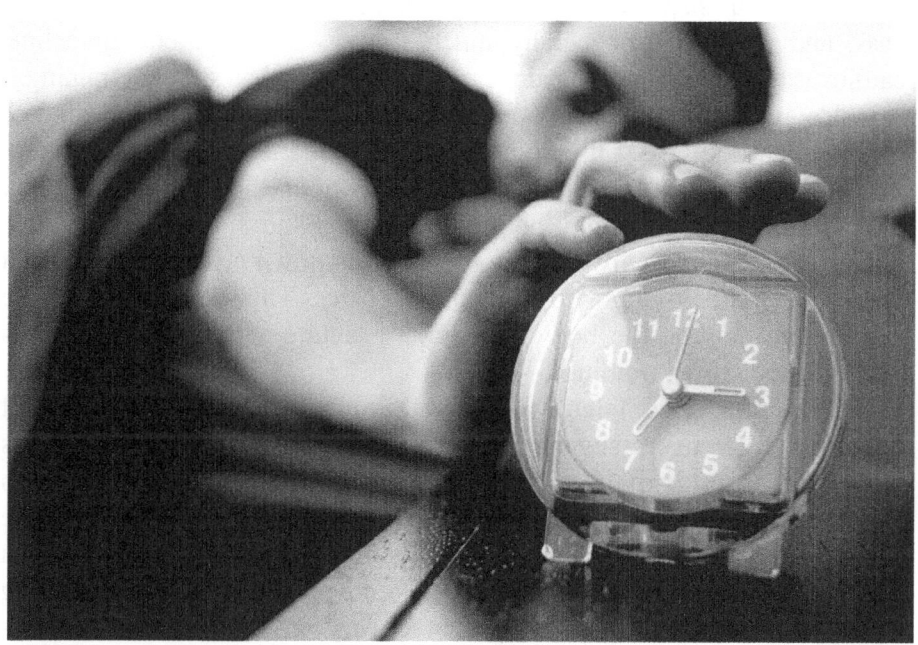

If rest and recovery are not sufficient, your body may adopt a permanently injured state and will not improve or adapt to the exercise. Hence, it is important to remember to allow adequate recovery between exercise sessions. This can sometimes be the reason why some people get mediocre results for the effort put in. It can be very difficult, however, to determine what 'sufficient' time is.

As a means to educate people, I came up with the 'black eye theory'. This theory explains what damage is caused when we strength train. It may help you in determining your 'sufficient' time and understand some of the issues that arise from strength training when you do not allow your body to sufficiently recover. With insufficient recovery similar damage could occur to your muscle fibers, tendons, ligaments, and stress hormones as though you sustained a black eye. The harder you train, the longer it takes to fully recuperate, not to mention, allowing your body to repair and super compensate (super compensation can be explained by when the muscle tissue has completely recovered and adapted to the applied stress placed upon it). Without adequate recovery, and pre-maturely resuming training, you could in fact cause more damage, which in turn, can make muscle gains dormant and increase the chance of injury. I recommend strength training 3 or 4 times per 7 - 8 days and as a general guideline strength training every second day, with a complete rest for approximately 7 days every 6 weeks of training. Cardiovascular training can be thought of as, instead of a black eye, more of a 'slap across the face.' Damage is still present but will soon pass, and recovery is generally much faster, - As a general guideline, cardiovascular training can be done more frequently than strength training.

Delayed-onset muscle soreness (doms) can occur after any kind of exercise, particularly if the body is in an unconditioned state relative to that exercise. Making sure you cool down and consume sufficient nutrition after training may help reduce doms and significantly reduce recovery time. Try to always take time to cool down properly. Aim for at least 10 minutes of light to medium intensity. This will help increase circulation, helping the body rid itself of lactate and metabolic wastes accumulated whilst training.

Once you've completely finished training, it is extremely important to refill the glycogen (sugar) stores in the muscles and liver. As long as you refuel your body (but being careful not to over-do it, this also depends on total basal metabolic rate and goals), recovery can take place, reducing soreness and hormonal stress. After exercise, there is a 30-45 minute window critical to muscle recovery. Before doing anything else, you should drink something for recovery. There are several studies provided by Dr John Ivy and Dr Robert Portman (The Performance Zone) that show high-glycemic carbohydrates (e.g, organic rice milk) and whey protein isolate (protein supplement) as being the most effective recovery beverage. It's ideal ratio can be seen as a 4:1 combination, an example would be 400 ml of organic rice milk equaling 40 grams of high-glycemic carbohydrates to 10 grams or whey protein isolate. Sports supplements like creatine, L-glutamine and magnesium are also recommended for exercise recovery. This particular nutrition advice is for anyone that has trained and depleted muscle glycogen storage. Drinking these 'refueling' supplements also helps to repair torn muscle fibers, reduce hormonal stress, increase muscle mass, improve metabolism, and decrease body fat.

Chapter Five

WHICH EXERCISES WILL REWARD ME THE MOST?

Compound Exercises vs Isolated Exercises
Compound exercises can be defined as any exercises that involves more than one joint and that usually activates more muscle groups and fibers than one muscle group. Isolated exercises are those that target single-joint actions or are prescribed to isolate individual muscles.

Compound exercises are effectively 'killing two birds with one stone'. Compound exercises increase metabolism and increase natural hormones like grow hormone and testosterone more than isolation exercises. Compound exercises should provide at least 80 per cent of your exercise selection in your strength-training program.

Why Compound? - Compound exercises are more functional to life.

Compound exercises:

Increase ability to safely lift heavy loads (which in turn activates more muscle for far better results)

Increased neurological activation (signaling from the brain to the muscle fibers themselves)

Increased muscle activation

Increased hormonal response

Increased basal metabolic rate

Promotes more joint stability

Incorporates the smaller muscles and at the same time reducing overall time in the gym.

Listed below are my top five favourite compound exercises for each major muscle group. They can be used for the basis of your strength-training program. These exercises have also been shown to activate the highest amount or muscle fibres.

CHEST	BACK	LEGS	TRICEPS	BICEPS	SHOULDERS
35° Incline Dumbbell Press	Wide-Grip Chin-up	Leg Press	Dips	Chin-ups	Standing Dumbbell Press
Flat Dumbbell Press	Lat Pull Down	Barbell Squat	Close-Grip Bench Press	Suprinated Lat Pull Down	Standing Barbell Press
Barbell Bench Press	Seated Row	Hack Squat	Straight Bar Standing Pushdowns	Straight Bar Standing Curls	
Standing Cable Fly	One Arm Dumbbell Row	Stationary Barbell Lunge	Close-Grip Push-ups	45° Seated Dumbbell Curls	
35° Incline Dumbbell Fly	Barbell Bent-Over Row	Step-ups			

Please note: Deadlifts recruit all muscle groups within the body and don't specifically recruit one particular bundle of muscle fibers. Deadlifts are classed as a compound exercise and would be one of the best exercises for all-a-round strength and conditioning. Deadlifts should be included in your routine, as should most Olympic power lifts and any human movement exercises that mimic daily movements. I also recommend mixing training schedule using the 'cross-fit' style training method. Visit www.crossfit.com for more information.

Varying speed of the exercise, changing muscle groups, selecting different exercises, and varying times and days that you work out will allow you to use these exercises for plenty of years to come.

Please note: To help understanding the exercises shown above I recommend the book 'Strength Training Anatomy' authored by Frederic Delavier.

I have included some sample balanced exercise programs using compound exercises.

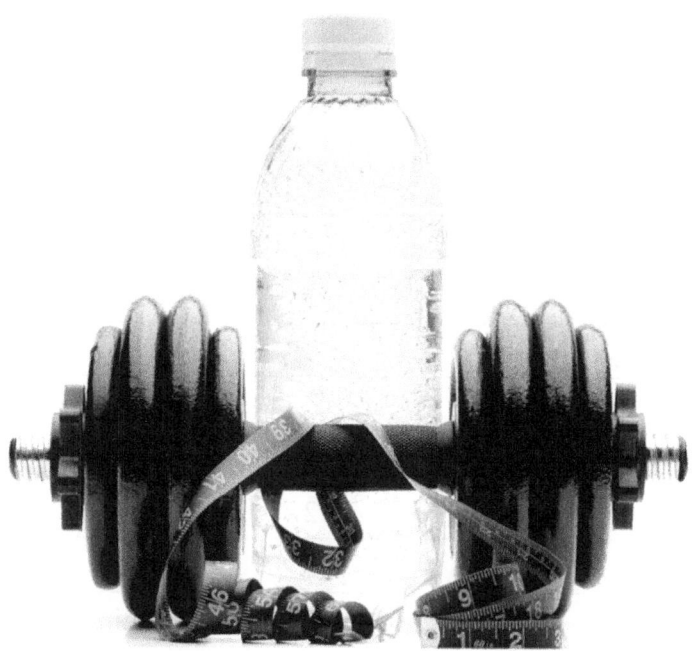

Sample exercise programs

Beginner Program - Full-body, two times per week.(e.g, Monday and Thursday)

MONDAY & THURSDAY	Total Sets	Total Reps
Warm up 3 - 5 minutes		
Bench Press	2 - 3	12 - 15
Seated Row	2 - 3	12 - 15
Leg Press	2 - 3	12 - 15
Assisted Dips	1 - 2	12 - 15
Assisted Chin-ups	1 - 2	12 - 15
Standing Shoulder Press	1 - 2	12 - 15
CARDIO = 20 minutes		
Heart Rate	130 to 140 beats per minute	
Type	Anything you like	

Intermediate program – Split program three times per week.
E.g. Monday, Wednesday and Friday

UPPER BODY	Total Sets	Total Reps
Warm Up 3 to 5 minutes		
35' Dumbbell Press	2 - 3	8 - 12
Lat Pull Down	2 - 3	8 - 12
Flat Dumbbell Fly	2 - 3	8 - 12
1 Arm Rows	2 - 3	8 - 12
Tricep Pushdowns	2 - 3	8 - 12
Standing Bicep Curls	2 - 3	8 - 12
CARDIO = 30 minutes		
Heart Rate	130 to 150 beats per minute	
Type	Anything you like	

LOWER BODY & CORE	Total Sets	Total Reps
Warm Up 3 to 5 minutes		
Leg Press	2 - 3	8 - 12
Stationary Lunges	2 - 3	8 - 12
Hack Squat	2 - 3	8 - 12
Pilates Plank	2 - 3	8 - 12
Reverse Crunch	2 - 3	8 - 12
CARDIO = 30 minutes		
Heart Rate	130 to 150 beats per minute	
Type	Anything you like	

FULL BODY	Total Sets	Total Reps
Warm Up 3 to 5 minutes		
35' Dumbbelll Press	2 - 3	8 - 12
Lat Pull Down	2 - 3	8 - 12
Leg Press	2 - 3	8 - 12
Push Ups	2 - 3	8 - 12
Box Jumps	2 - 3	8 - 12
CARDIO = 30 minutes		
Heart Rate	130 to 150 beats per minute	
Type	Anything you like	

Advanced program – Split program four days per week.

E.g. First week Monday, Wednesday, Friday and Sunday

Second week Tuesday, Thursday, Saturday and Monday and so on.

CHEST & BICEPS	Total Sets	Total Reps
Warm Up 3 to 5 minutes		
Standing Cable Fly's	2 - 3	6 - 8
35' Dumbbell Press	2 - 3	6 - 8
Bench Press	2 - 3	6 - 8
Weighted Chin Ups	2 - 3	6 - 8
Seated Dumbbell Curls	2 - 3	6 - 8
CARDIO = 30 minutes – Interval Sprints		
Heart Rate	130 to 160 beats per minute	
Type	Anything you like	

LEGS & CORE	Total Sets	Total Reps
Warm Up 3 to 5 minutes		
Weighted Step Ups	2 - 3	6 - 8
Squats	2 - 3	6 - 8
Single Leg-Leg Press	2 - 3	6 - 8
Deadlifts	2 - 3	6 - 8
Pilates Rocks	2 - 3	15 - 20
Hanging Leg Raises	2 - 3	15 - 20
CARDIO = 30 minutes – Interval Sprints		
Heart Rate	130 to 160 beats per minute	
Type	Anything you like	

BACK & TRICEPS	Total Sets	Total Reps
Warm Up 3 to 5 minutes		
Seated Row	2 - 3	6 - 8
Wide Grip Chin Ups	2 - 3	6 - 8
BB Bent Over Row	2 - 3	6 - 8
Weighted Dips	2 - 3	6 - 8
Close Grip Bench Press	2 - 3	6 - 8
CARDIO = 30 minutes – Interval Sprints		
Heart Rate	130 to 150 beats per minute	
Type	Anything you like	

300 Cross-fit Style	Total Sets	Total Reps
Warm Up 3 to 5 minutes		
Chin Ups	1	25

300 Cross-fit Style	Total Sets	Total Reps
Dumbbell Deadlifts	1	50
Push Ups	1	50
Box Jumps	1	50
Abdominal wipers	1	50
1 Arm Dumbbell Snatch	1	25 each arm
Chin Ups	1	25
CARDIO = 30 minutes		
Heart Rate	130 to 160 beats per minute	
Type	Anything you like	

300 Cross-fit workout please note: Beginners use bodyweight

Intermediate use 15-25% of body weight

Advanced 25-50% of body weight

For example: If I was intermediate and weighed 100kgs.

I would use 15-25 kg Dumbbells when performing the Dumbbell Deadlifts.

Chapter Six

THE DANGER ZONE: HOW TO AVOID INJURIES

Too often, a person will choose a strength-training exercise program that has been passed down from prior generations rather than choosing one based on proven, scientific, safe, and time-efficient principles. More often than not, injuries occur when either picking up the weight or when setting the weight back. Be sure to always use correct form when picking up or putting back the weight. Other causes for injuries are by poor technique, lifting weights too heavy or executing an exercise that is too advanced for your training age. The following list provides exercises that can potentially cause injury and need NOT be included in your strength training program. These exercises one way or another have been proven to add little benefit whilst adding a high risk of injury. You will never see an educated trainer prescribing any of the following exercises. Using compound exercises will ensure all muscles will have been targeted and strengthened.

"No matter what, avoid the following exercises.'

1. Chest Pec Deck with no adjustment
2. Decline Bench Press
3. Behind the Neck Shoulder Press
4. Behind the Neck Lat Pull Down
5. Pullovers
6. Upright Rows
7. Dumbbell Lateral and Front Raises
8. Shrugs
9. Overhead Tricep Extensions

10. Roman Chair Back Extensions

11. Stiff Legged Dead lifts

12. Good Mornings

13. Leg Extensions

14. Hamstring Leg Curls.

Understanding Safety and Perfect Posture

When we execute an exercise it is extremely important to understand how to stand and move. Some exercises are performed standing up, seated, some are done lying down while others are done moving. Good form indicates the following body postures.

Standing setup:
- Feet hip width apart
- Knees slightly bent
- Pelvis square and neutral
- Abdominals engaged
- Shoulders retracted and down
- Looking forward with slight chin tuck
- Breathing out at the hardest part of the exercise

For seated setup:
- Adjust seat (where possible) so that knees are slightly below hip height
- Feet hip width apart
- Pelvis square and neutral
- Abdominals engaged
- Shoulders retracted and down
- Looking forward with slight chin tuck
- Breathing out at the hardest part of the exercise

When moving setup:
- Pelvis square and neutral
- Abdominals engaged
- Shoulders retracted and down
- Looking forward with slight chin tuck
- Breathing out at the hardest part of the exercise

Other things to consider:
- Always use the Valsalva Maneuver - Simply put; breathe out at the hardest part of the movement. This will ensure control and tightening of the abdominal muscles to protect the spine and lower back.
- Always protect your back – When correct technique is performed the hip line will be slightly higher than that of the rest of the body.

Chapter Seven

ADVANCED SIMPLICITY

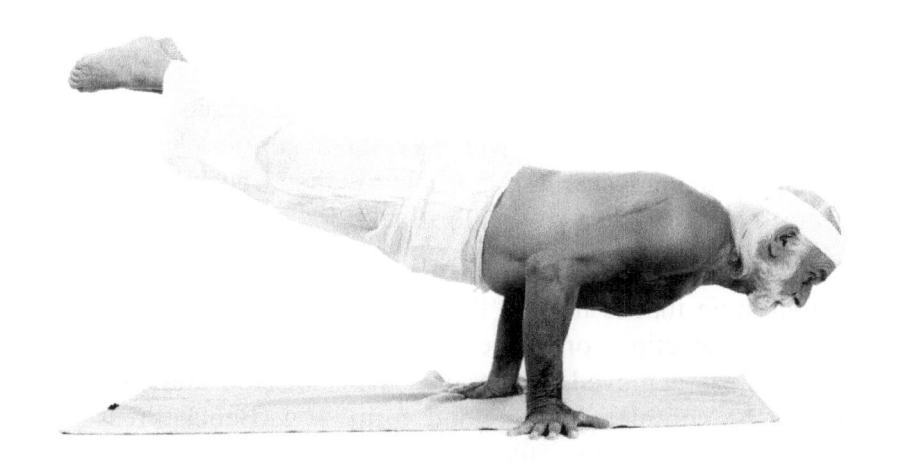

For those who have been training for some time you may need and like to mix it up. Challening your body is a great means for continued growth. The following techniques can be used by those who have excellent control and strength. Who has also mastered the correct breathing techniques. All of these training styles are intermediate to advanced and should only be completed if you have been training for at least a year.

Superset – Executing an exercise using the same muscle group but going from one exercise to another with little to no rest.

E.g. Bench Press to Dumbbell Fly to Pushups then rest. This can also be also done using different muscles groups. E.g. Bench Press (chest) then Seated Row (back)

Drop set – Executing the same exercise starting with the heaviest weight and dropping the weight till no reps can be completed with perfect posture. E.g. Bench Press 100kg for 6 reps then drop weight to 90kgs for

6 reps dropping to 80kgs for 6 reps then resting or until no reps can be done with good form.

Eccentrics – When performing eccentric training always use a well educated spotter. This particular training style is in my eyes the most advanced of all training and can challenge even the most experienced strength trainer. Eccentric training is referred as the down phase of the repetition. You would need to increase the weight by approximately 15-20% above what they would normally lift in both up and down phases. Now your aim here is to control only the down phase and your spotter will help lift the weight back up. Aim to control the down movement for 4 to 6 seconds and repeat for between 6-10 reps.

Pre-exhausting – This advanced principle is designed to execute an isolation exercise first followed by a compound exercise focusing on the same muscle grouping. This will cause the major muscles to work harder to complete the movement. E.g. Cable Fly then Bench Press for Chest or Reverse Fly's then Seated Row for Back.

HITT (high intensity type training) – This is a high intensity training style that is not for the faint at heart. Similar to a drop set. HITT is selecting one exercise and continuing until complete exhaustion is achieved. The trainer will not stop until not one more rep can be completed with good form. E.g. Bench Press 100kg to 90kg to 80kg to 60kg to 50kg to 30kg to the bar to pushups.

Repetition ranges for optimal growth and metabolism change

Although the exact stimulus for muscle growth is still not 100% known, research from Dr Mauro Di Pasquale supports one or more of the following factors must take place.

1. High tension training (heavy loading)
2. Metabolic work (compound exercises)
3. Eccentric muscle actions (down phase of lifting)
4. Hormonal response to training.

Here is a list of what different repetition numbers have on training stimulus.

Rep Range	Primary Adaption	Energy Used
1-4	Neural improvement	Creatinephosphate
4-6	Growth of Type2b fibers	Glycogen/Lactic Acid
6-20	Growth of Type2a fibers	Glycogen/Lactic Acid
20-30	Increased sarcoplasmic volume	Glycogen/Fat/Protein

Irrespective of the above factors, the ultimate key to larger and stronger muscles is progressive overload. This means each and every time you are in the gym training you should be trying to achieve either a higher weight or complete more reps that you previously completed. This can be achieved by following some simple rules.

These include: using a weight between 60-85% of maximal, using controlled eccentric (lowering) movements, applying proper progressive overload principles (increasing load when allotted number of reps are completed), adequate recovery nutrition, allowing adequate rest and recovery and only training a particular muscle group once every 4-7 days.

Interesting fact: Studies show muscle growth occurs when Type 2 fibers are stimulated (6-20 reps).

Chapter Eight

CARDIOVASCULAR EXERCISE

The American College of Sports Medicine (ACSM) and the American Heart Association (AHA) released updated physical activity guidelines in 2007. The ACSM and the AHA suggests that people should engage in continuous cardiovascular activity for at least 30 to 60 minutes 3 to 5 times every week. This can include anything that you enjoy that will increase resting heart rate. This activity creates a stronger and more efficient heart and lungs and effectively increases circulation. If you are new to exercising, for your safety, I encourage the use of your maximum heart rate zoning guidelines (see table below). These guidelines will determine if you are working appropriately enough for continued results and more importantly, making sure you are not training too intensely.

Training Heart Rate Zones	
Determine your maximum training heart rate (MHR)	
220 subtract your age = MHR	
Beginner Trainer	55% - 65% of your maximum
Intermediate Trainer	65% - 75% of your maximum
Advanced Trainer	75% - 85% of your maximum

Using a heart rate monitor is an awesome way of determining this level.

Cardiovascular timing for a better fat burning effect

Exercising timing for fat loss can make or break your overall result. Morning exercise before eating can produce more fat used as energy since your body is in a hypoglycemic (low on sugar in the blood) state as mention in earlier chapters. Your body will have a tendency to use far more fat as fuel. Any type of cardiovascular exercise is suggested. If exercising in the morning is too inconvenient, consider strength training before your cardiovascular training. This will help breakdown glycogen storage therefore forcing your body to use more stored energy from fat stores when cardiovascular training commences. As a general rule of thumb, cardiovascular exercise should last no longer than 60 minutes in a completely carbohydrate depleted state.

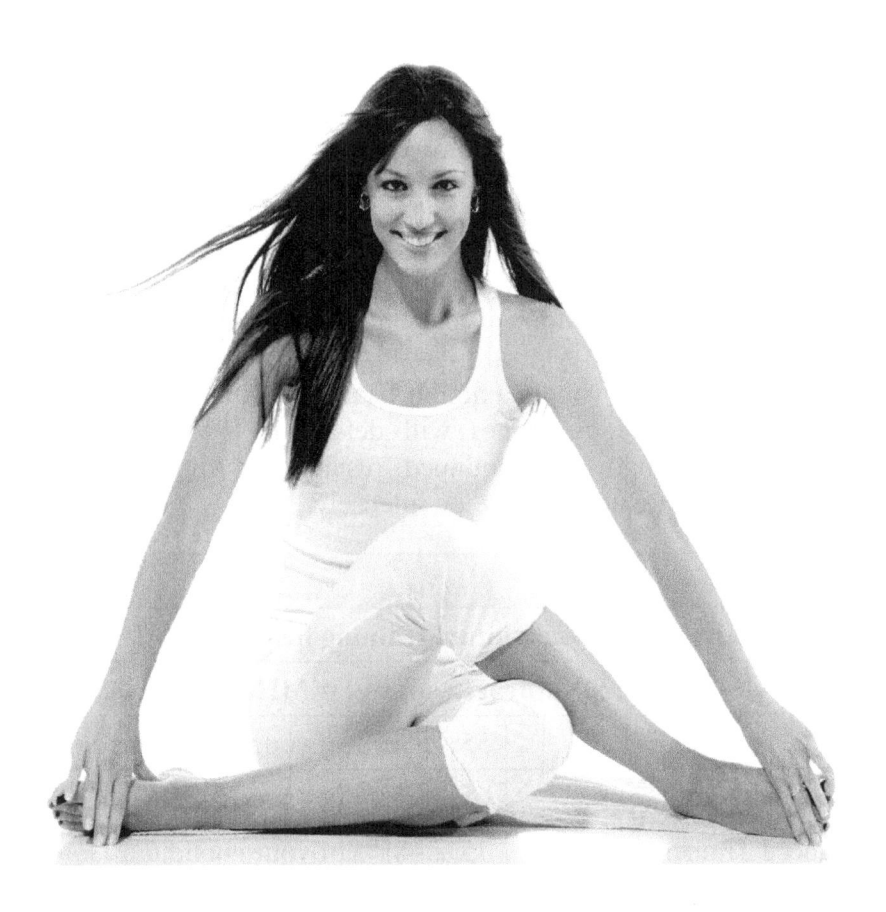

Chapter Nine

FLEXIBILITY

Long, lean, flexible muscles will guard against injury whether you are at work, rest or play. Flexibility and strength are critical in life and are key components to all successful athletes and competitors. If you stretch, you will live longer – Period!

Stretch and relaxation programs, such as, yoga, pilates, and Tai Chi will help blood circulation and improve overall quality of life. Even stretching after your workout helps in this regard. I also recommend that combining a light cardiovascular cool down, no longer than 10 minutes, not increasing heart rate higher than 120bpm will improve muscle damage and increase recovery rates.

This time will also allow you to de-stress your mind and enjoy exercise without strenuous pressure. The brain is a major part of what we stretch when we do stretching exercises. Connective tissue is injured when we exercise. Stretching can also help lower cortisol hormone. Although rich in nerves, connective tissue has a poor blood supply, particularly at the junctions with the bone and muscle. When light stretching force is applied, the tendons, ligaments, muscles and bones are separated slightly which will allow an increase in blood flow to nourish affected areas. Take time out and positively stretch each major muscle grouping 2 to 3 times per week. A great book – 'The Anatomy of Stretching' by Brad Walker will help with your stretching techniques

Major benefits of flexibility training

- ✓ Increased circulation
- ✓ Increase range of motion (making you more agile and will help reduce the chance of injury)
- ✓ Increased muscle strength
- ✓ Reduced muscle tension

- ✓ Reduced muscle soreness
- ✓ Reduced muscle spasms
- ✓ Enhanced healing of microscopic muscle fiber tears
- ✓ Enhanced relaxation
- ✓ Enhanced posture
- ✓ Decrease in stress hormone cortisol

Part Two

Nutrition

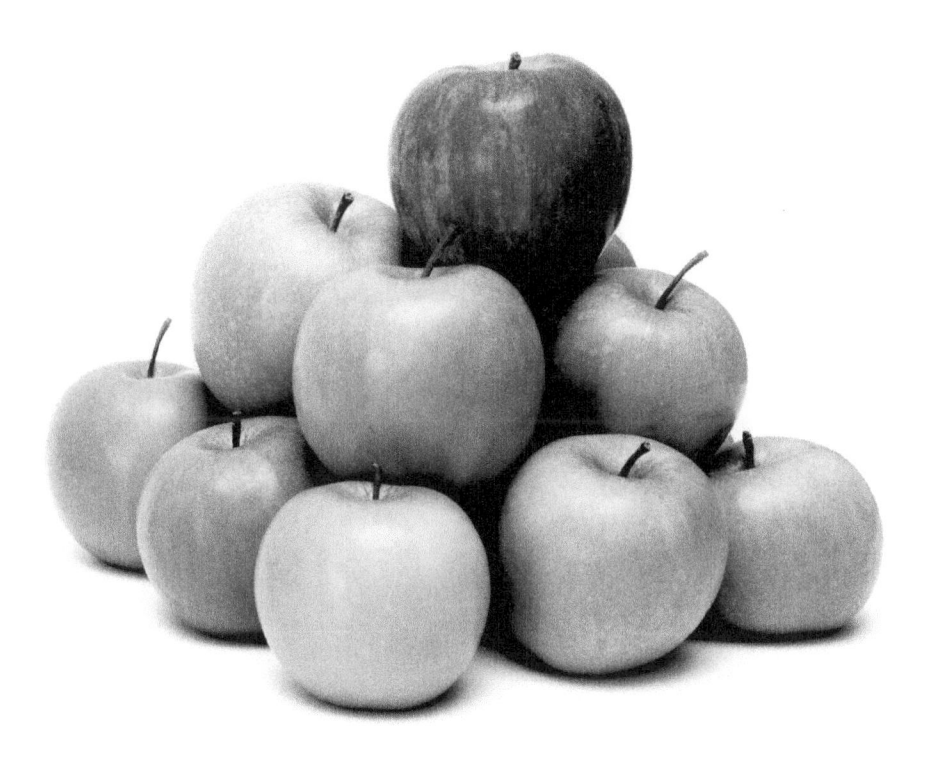

Good nutritional habits are now more important to your health and fat loss as exercise. When exercising, it is just as important to have a good balanced nutrition plan to ensure that the body has the correct amount of carbohydrates, protein & fat (macro-nutrients). This will insure the body has the best chance to help the recovery process following hard exercise and work sessions.

Chapter Ten

40:30:30 – GET IN THE ZONE

But what is the correct ratio of macro-nutrients?

Why are people having some much trouble losing weight?

The food pyramid that has been promoted for more than 40 years is based upon guidelines suggested by the US Department of Health (USDH). This ratio is Carbohydrates 60%, Protein 15% and Fats 25%. You might be surprised to learn, however, that the United States Department of Agriculture (USDA), not the Health Department, conducted the research and set these guidelines. In that way, the guidelines pertain more to fattening cattle than to providing proper nutrition to humans. Think about it. People who follow the food pyramid are following a nutrition plan that fattens up livestock in the shortest amount of time. Why do that? David Kritchevsky – The Wistar Institute (Philadelphia USA) cited in the JN-The Journal of Nutrition that 'In the late 1950's, the US government established the link between heart disease and saturated fat.'

They told the American public to cut fat from their diets and in its place eat more carbohydrates. They suggested if you did this, not only would the rate of heart disease decrease but so would obesity, which in fact also started to increase. In 1955, studies prove that 40% of our calories came from fat, in 1992, only 35%. Sadly, however, our obesity increased rather than decreased. The statistics are startling.

In 1962, 23% of the population was obese. In 1990 it had increased to 35%. The American Diabetic Association conducted research reported that between the 1970's and the 1980's obesity increased by over 30%, fat intake dropped by around 10% and even total calories decreased by an average of 5% but yet society still gained bodyweight. Remember, we were originally told to eat less fat and more carbohydrates, now these studies prove that this ratio was not helping obesity and not maintaining optimal health.

The ratio of 40% Carbohydrates, 30% Protein and 30% Healthy Fat not only help's us maintain optimal weight but optimal health. We need a good mix of every macro-nutrient to survive and by following this ratio, it will help create easy lifestyle choices that will leave you full-filled, content and most importantly not depriving your body's needs.

40 % CARBOHYDRATES
30 % PROTEIN
30 % FAT

Chapter Eleven

INSULIN AND GLUCAGON

Insulin just like metabolism, is known by all of us, but very few have a good understanding of what it is and why it's so important! Insulin whilst being very complex is also very simple. Insulin is a hormone that has effects on metabolism and other body functions. Insulin causes cells in the liver, muscle, and fat tissue to take up glucose from the blood stream, storing it as glycogen in the liver and muscle, and stopping use of fat as an energy source. When insulin is low, glucose is not taken up by body cells, and the body begins to use fat as an energy source. Insulin is also classed as an 'anabolic' hormone and is a key component to recovery as it signals the body for repair and growth. Without insulin, amino acid (digested protein) uptake within muscle cells will cease. Insulin is produced in the pancreas and released when different types of food or drink, such as ingested protein and carbohydrates, are consumed. The insulin is released to take up the glucose produced from these foods and drinks. Not all types of carbohydrate produce glucose and thereby increase blood glucose levels but most do. "Here's one way to think about it. Think of a can of regular soft drink (a high-glycemic, refined, simple carbohydrate) as petrol for your body (your car). Now think of insulin as the petrol pump, pumping the petrol in your fuel tank. You would never get 15 petrol pumps and try filling your car's fuel tank all at the same time. You would also never try and fill your tank with 100 litres of fuel if you only had a 60 litre tank. When you consume too much high-glycemic, refined, simple carbohydrates, far too much insulin is excreted fast, taking the sugar from your blood stream and delivering it into the liver, muscles and fat. The body simply cannot utilise that amount of fuel at that particular time. Low and medium glycemic carbohydrates are like using one petrol pump, slowly pumping fuel into your fuel tanks. To help maintain insulin levels, always consume protein and some fat with any type of carbohydrates.

Glucagon is the reason why I suggest exercising first thing in the morning or when you are in a carbohydrate depleted state. Glucagon is also an important hormone involved in carbohydrate metabolism. Produced by the pancreas also, it is released when blood glucose levels decline, this causing the liver to convert stored glycogen into glucose (sugar) and release it into the bloodstream. This helps raise blood glucose levels and ultimately preventing the development of low blood sugar. The action of glucagon is opposite to that of insulin. Glucagon helps maintain the level of glucose via the liver, releasing glucose (through a process known as glycogenolysis). This glucose is released into the bloodstream. Both of these mechanisms lead to glucose release by the liver. Glucagon also regulates the rate of glucose production through lipolysis (fat burning). Simply put, when you are carbohydrate depleted your body is forced by a complex number of chemical reactions to draw glucose from storage and use it as energy. Utilising this hormone is critical to fast and constant fat loss. Insulin pushes glucose and nutrients into the cells, whilst glucagon takes glucose and nutrients from the cells. Because of the competing nature of insulin and glucagon, building muscle and burning fat usually cannot be accomplished at the same time. Here's why. Insulin is anabolic (rebuilding) and glucagon is catabolic (breaking down). This is extremely difficult (but is not impossible) to manipulate them together for muscle growth whilst using fat as energy. This may explain why professional body builder's cycle calories from season to season. If your goal is muscle building then you need to use insulin frequently by consuming carbohydrates and if your goal is fat loss you must train in a carbohydrate depleted state. The key to decreasing fat storage and increasing lean muscle at the same time can be achieved by mimicking these hormones by cycling calories from day to day. Using low calories on training days and high calories on resting days.

Chapter Twelve

CARBOHYDRATES

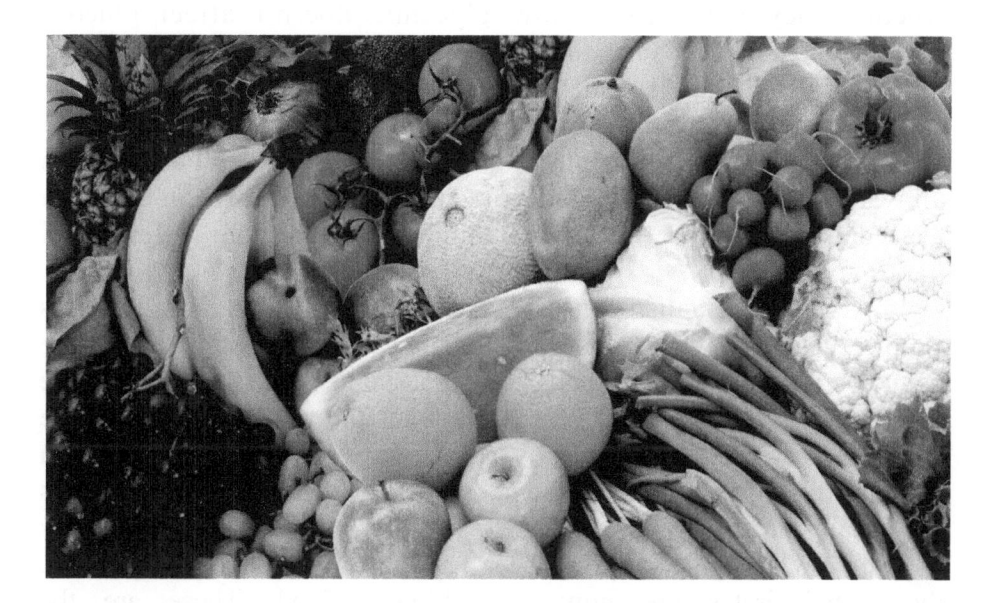

Carbohydrates are the **major source of energy** for muscular exertion and aid in digestion and assimilation of all foods. Carbohydrates when digested are broken down into blood sugar or glucose and combined with water to form glycogen that is stored in muscle cells and our liver. Excess glucose is stored in the fat cells throughout the body as a reserve source of energy. Glycogen is the primary fuel for muscle contraction. As you can now see if we over eat carbohydrates (especially refined and high glycemic carbohydrates) the more glucose will be stored.

Carbohydrates are present in foods in the forms of simple and complex composition. The difference pertains to the rate at which the food is broken down into blood glucose and pushed into the liver, muscle cells and or stored in fat cells. If a food causes rapid rise in blood glucose, then it referred as "high glycemic" and one that causes slow blood glucose is referred as "low glycemic". The glycemic index is a scientific tested index of all food and liquids and the speed in which they are broken down into glucose.

A number of factors affect the glycemic index of a carbohydrate. This includes chemical composition, amount of fiber, protein or fat contained in the food and how the food is cooked or prepared. Remember though, it isn't just the rate of glucose entering the bloodstream that dictates how much will be converted into body fat but also the amount of carbohydrates consumed. By using the 40:30:30 macro-nutrients guidelines the selection of carbohydrates whether they are high or low glycemic doesn't affect glucose storage as much because fats and proteins slow the absorption of glucose into the cells. Therefore making sure that the particular carbohydrate you have selected gets absorbed slowly and limits the chance to completely saturate muscle cells and liver. This method allows us to select high and low glycemic carbohydrates as an everyday choice and this helps maintain optimal energy levels all the time.

A typical Australian consumes about 60% of their carbohydrates as simple sugars. Which are added to foods rather than those that come naturally in fruits and vegetables. These simple sugars come in large amounts in soft drinks and fast food. Over the course of a year, the average Australian consumes over 100 litres of soft drinks, which contains the highest amount of added sugars. Even though carbohydrates are usually necessary for humans to function, they are not all equally healthful. When machinery has been used to remove bits of high fiber, the carbohydrates are now classed as refined. These are the carbohydrates found in white bread and fast food. I urge you to limit refined carbohydrates and simple sugars to make sure your carbohydrates are absorbed slowly into your bloodstream.

Most food labels are written in kilojoules, this has been suggested as a means to confuse the consumer in hope you still decide to consume it. Simply divide kilojoules by 4 to get an approximate amount of calories. The amount of calories you need in a day reflects your basal metabolic rate, lifestyle and exercise expenditure.

Reading the labels

Make sure you check the carbohydrate to sugar ratio on the nutritional label.

Nutrition Facts

Serving Size 1 slice (47g)
Servings Per Container 6

Amount Per Serving	
Calories 160	Calories from Fat 90
	% Daily Value*
Total Fat 10g	15%
Saturated Fat 2.5g	11%
Trans Fat 2g	
Cholesterol 0mg	0%
Sodium 300mg	12%
Total Carb 15g	5%
Dietary Fiber less than 1g	3%
Sugars 1g	
Protein 3g	

Vitamin A 0%	Vitamin C 4%
Calcium 45%	Iron 6%
Thiamin 8%	Riboflavin 6%
Niacin 6%	

*Percent Daily Values are based on a 2,000 calorie diet. Your daily values may be higher or lower depending on your calorie needs.

Start here

Check the total calories per serving

Limit these nutrients

Get enough of these nutrients

Quick Guide to % Daily Value:
5% or less is low
20% or more is high

- ✓ This example: Total carbohydrate = 15 grams
- ✓ Total sugars = 1 gram

For the typical gym junkie trying to pack on extra muscle tissue, carbohydrate overloading can overload your system which can cause chronic insulin response and decrease the 2 critical hormones needed for optimal muscle growth – testosterone and growth hormone. Higher carbohydrates can also increase the level of serotonin, a chemical in the brain that can make you tired, relaxed and ready for sleep. It can also make you retain more fluid as one gram of refined sugar equals three grams water held. It can also leave you feeling bloated and uncomfortable.

By simply reducing your consumption of carbohydrates, especially refined carbohydrates, and replacing them with good, essential fats, you will reduce your body fat, increase natural hormones, reduce fluid retention, and keep your energy level high and stable all day long. This will also ensure full recovery and optimal muscle growth. To build muscle you must consume plenty of essential fatty acids like flaxseed oil, olive oil and some saturated fats like in organic rump steak and coconut oils. This helps to reconstruct hormones needed for muscle growth and aid in reducing inflammation of the joints.

1 GRAM OF CARBOHYDRATES = 4 CALORIES

CARBOHYDRATES DO NOT MAKE YOU FAT

OVER EATING REFINED AND SIMPLE CARBOHYDRATES WILL MAKE YOU FAT

Chapter Thirteen

PROTEIN

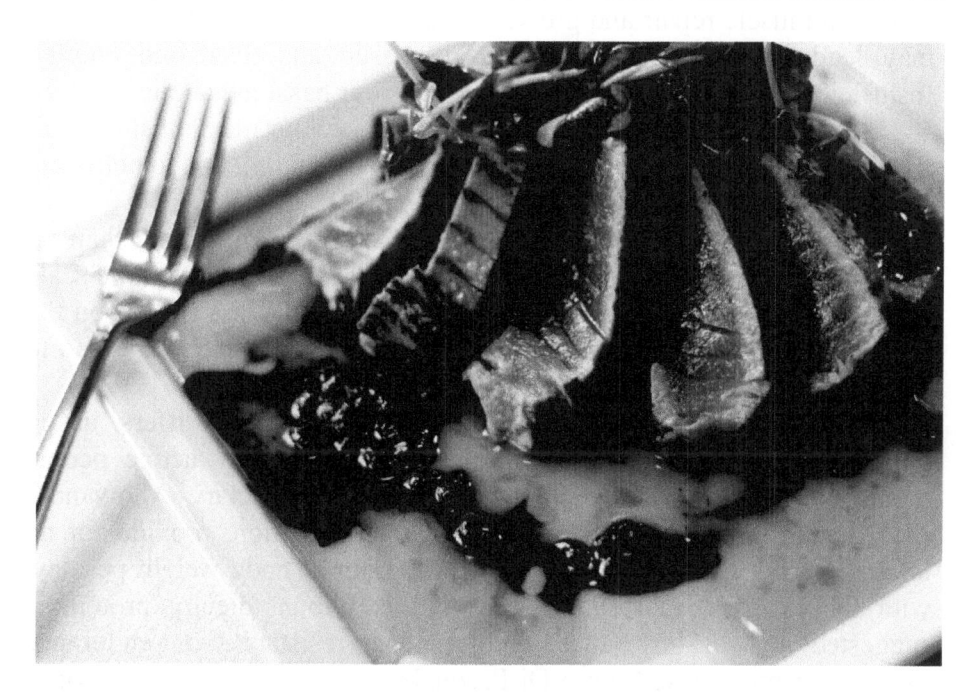

Protein feeds the muscle. Without sufficient protein, muscles cannot survive and will break down. Even if you are not exercising trying to developing new muscle tissue, you must supply protein to the muscles every day. Anyone that has severely dieted or restricted calories have no doubt lost important metabolic muscle. Most people cannot afford to lose any muscle tissue. Muscle is an active tissue, meaning it burns calories. The more muscle you have, the more calories your body will burn and the faster your metabolism will be. Proteins are the second most abundant substance in the body and are the building blocks for all cells. Protein's, when digested, are broken down into simple units called amino acids and are then synthesized by the body. The human body requires 22 amino acids and all but 8 can be produced by the body. These 8 are known as 'essential amino acids' and must be supplied by our own nutrition. Protein cannot be stored in the body which means supplying protein at different intervals everyday is essential.

Most meat, fish and dairy products are complete protein foods (meaning has all the amino acids needed for complete repair), whilst most fruit and vegetables are incomplete protein foods. The ultimate goal is to have a sufficient amount of amino acids creating a positive nitrogen balance. A positive nitrogen balance allows the body to be in an anabolic state (muscle's in an environment to repair and grow) that results in muscle repair and growth. If amino acids are in short supply it may lead to a breakdown in muscle tissue and decreased energy. Insufficient amino acids may also cause a lower basal metabolic rate.

Consume protein at every meal to increase your metabolism, repair tissue, slow carbohydrate response, to help you feel full, and to help curb sugar cravings.

Remember that muscle can weigh up to three times more than fat but usually takes up half the space. This means more weight on the scale but creating half the belt size. Loss of muscle means less weight on the scale however less muscle means slower metabolism which may lead to easy body fat gain.

The protein requirement for each individual does differs, as do opinions about whether and to what extent physically active people require more protein. The 2005 Recommended Dietary Allowances (RDA), aimed at the general healthy adult population, provide for an intake of 0.8 - 1 grams of protein per kilogram of body weight per day, with the review panel stating that "no additional dietary protein is suggested for healthy adults undertaking resistance or endurance exercise'. Conversely, Mauro Di Pasquale (2008), assistant professor at the University of Toronto Canada and author of the 'Anabolic Diet' citing recent studies, recommends a minimum protein intake of 2.2 g/kg "for anyone involved in competitive or intense recreational sports who wants to maximize lean body mass but does not wish to gain weight."

Unfortunately the common fitness participant (usually males) over consumes protein intake in the hope that they will develop bigger larger denser muscle tissue which in fact is not true. This excess protein intake can contribute to a larger amount of energy stored as fat due to the fact that over half ingested protein is converted as glucose, raising insulin. Therefore as so many experts state, 1.5 grams protein x body weight is all the protein required for the recreational trainer to maintain positive nitrogen balance. Doing so will optimise muscle growth and recovery. Another interesting factor about protein is that approximately 5-10% extra calories are burnt from eating protein as for carbohydrates even though gram for gram both equal the same. This is caused by the thermal effect to eating protein. E.g. 100 calories protein eaten = 20-25 calories extra burnt.

1 GRAM OF PROTEIN = 4 CALORIES

PROTEIN
DOES NOT MAKE YOU FAT

OVER EATING OR UNDER EATING PROTEIN WILL MAKE YOU FAT

Chapter Fourteen

FAT

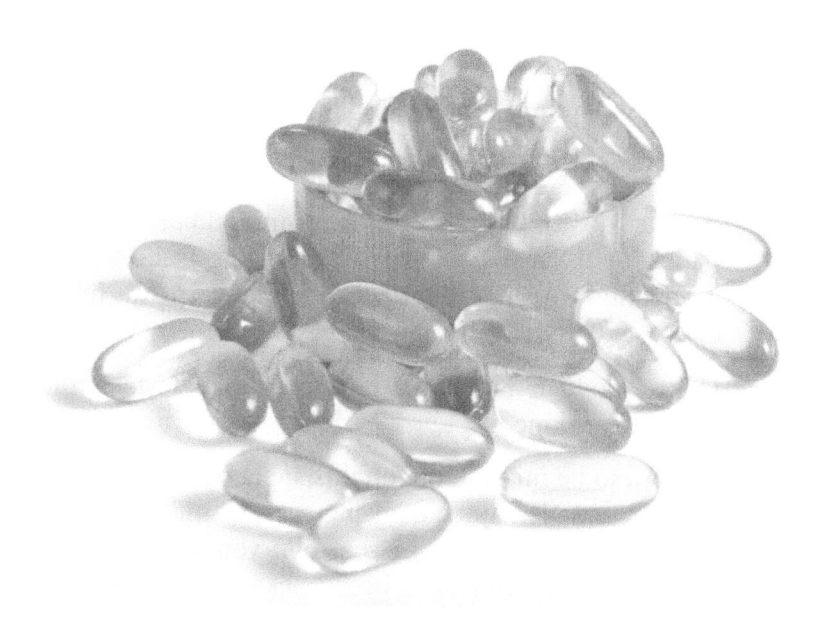

Without consuming adequate fats you will never experience optimal health. The foods we eat contain many different types of fats, and the building blocks of these fats are known as fatty acid molecules. A drop of olive oil contains a billion fatty acid molecules. The important thing though, is that some of these fatty acids are absolutely essential for life and optimal health, some are non-essential and some positively harmful.

To simplify things, you can think of the fatty acids in your diet as falling into one of three categories.

1 Essential, healthful fats
2 Neutral fats with no real health benefits
3 Harmful or killer fats.

The Natural Health Society in Australia estimates 90% of modern diets are low or deficient in the essential fats; some scientists believe that this is one of the greatest nutritional problems facing us. The benefit of consuming plenty of essential fatty acids (EFA's) is impressive to say the least.

Essential fatty acids contain numerous benefits. Here are some of them:

- Much-needed hydration for healthy skin and hair
- A huge role in immune function, helping to keep infection and colds at bay
- Crucial for brain development and well-being
- Needed to elevate mood and to lift depression
- Contributing to less sugar cravings and problem eating
- Increases energy and stamina but aids in recovery as well
- Appear to have powerful anti-inflammatory properties which helps speed wound healing, this is because of the lubrication of the joints. It also helps with lubricating congested bowels; this makes waste extremely easy to pass
- Helps produce important hormones like testosterone and growth hormone

Can you afford to be missing out on this super nutrient?

The top four essential fatty acids being flaxseed oil, hemp seed oil, pumpkin seed oil and walnuts. If you use seed oils, you must make sure that they are fresh; cold pressed and have been packaged in an oxygen free container. Look for polyunsaturated fats which consist of omega 3 and omega 6 fatty acids because these fatty acids can't be made by the body.

Killer fats lay at the root of much degenerated disease, such as cancer, heart disease and immune diseases because of it chemically unstable composition. These include any fats that include high saturated fat molecules like bacon, margarine and any source that has turned hard at room temperature. Saturated fats and cholesterol are often found together in a variety of foods including red meats, full cream milk, butter, sausages and most processed foods. Butter, cream and cheese are actually quite neutral in the body providing there are plenty of essential fatty acids present. Essential fatty acids have also been used by educated health professionals for years as an aid in lowering high cholesterol levels.

1 GRAM OF FAT = 9 CALORIES

FAT DOES NOT MAKE YOU FAT

OVER EATING OR UNDER EATING FAT WILL MAKE YOU FAT

Chapter Fifteen

WATER

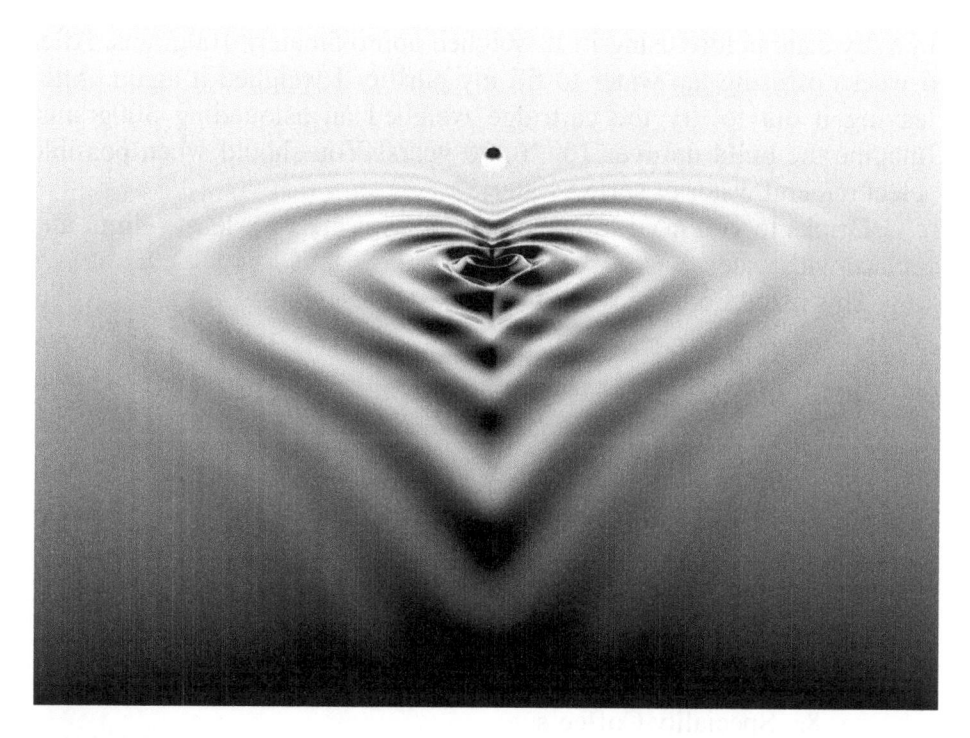

Water is one of the most important nutrients in the diet, if not the most. Water should be your number one choice when choosing what to drink. Water helps eliminate food waste products in the body, regulates body temperature during activity and helps with digestion. Maintaining hydration during periods of physical exertion is key to peak performance. While drinking too much water during activities can lead to physical discomfort, dehydration markedly hindered athletic performance.

If you consume too much water at any one given time your body may be forced to excrete more than needed leaving you more dehydrated than you first were. Drink smaller amounts slowly and often throughout the day especially before and during meals. As a general rule consume 1L (1000ml) or pure spring water for every 25kgs of body weight in each 24 hour period. Unfortunately studies are proving how bad our water is becoming in today's world. A study conducted by the US geological survey in 2002 (imagine what it would be today) found that over 80% of our water is contaminated by detergents, hormones like estrogen, anti-depressants, fecal matters, shampoos, chemicals like prozac, fluoride and literally thousands of micro-scopic particles. I conducted my own study here in my home. I purchased a 'Brita' water purifier that uses cartridge technology. I decided to weigh the cartridge in a dry state before using it. It weighed approximately 100grams. After 6 weeks of using tap water to fill my purifier I weighed it again. After leaving it out to dry the cartridge weighed an astounding 300grams. Imagine the build up over 10, 20, 30 years! You should when possible select mineral water or spring water.

Drinks to you need to leave behind or at the very least – limit and replace with water.

This list is from the worst to the least worse.

1. Soft Drinks
2. Energy Drinks
3. Diet Drinks (all)
4. Fruit Flavoured Alcohol
5. Alcohol
6. Fruit Flavoured Kids Drinks
7. Sports Drinks
8. Speciality Coffee's
9. Fruit Juices
10. Non-Organic Milk

The above drinks have proven to add little health and cause more harm than well intentioned. Without going into depth, these drinks one way or another slow cellular function, decrease metabolism, increase dehydration, steal important minerals, cause abnormalities like allergies and lead to a breeding ground for ill health.

Chapter Sixteen

BASAL METABOLIC RATE

Basal Metabolic Rate (BMR) can be defined as the amount of energy expended while at rest usually in a 24 hour period. The release of energy at rest is sufficient only for the functioning of the vital organs, such as the heart, lungs, brain, the nervous system, liver, kidneys, sex organs, muscles and skin. Without adequate calorie supply normal body function cannot exist. Key to easy fat loss and/or muscle gains depends on your particular BMR. BMR can usually decrease with age and is commonly due to the loss of lean muscle tissue. Increasing muscle mass increases basal metabolic rate. Any type of exercise can also increase basal metabolic rate. Strength training has been shown to be the most effective.

Without adequate calorie supply, (usually any calorie number below your basal metabolic rating) your body will go under huge stress, producing enzymes to preserve fat. This will cause a shift in calories used as energy and may mean protein (amino acids) may be used as the preferred energy choice. This can and no doubt lead to muscle loss. This is a well known term called 'starvation'. Our body slows basic normal bodily functions as a safely mechanism to save and preserve energy. Unfortunately any foods consumed whilst in this stage may be stored directly into fat cells.

Knowing your basal metabolic rate is more important than anyone ever gives credit for. This is another key component to extreme success. This can easily be tested using bio-impedance or MRI. After years of literally testing thousands of people, as a general guide, here is my basic basal metabolic rating's for both sexes.

	Basal Metabolic Rating
Females	1500 – 1800 calories per day
Males	1800 – 2200 calories per day

This would be the minimum total calorie consumption for any individual looking to reduce body fat, keep homeostasis (normal balanced body functions and hormones) and maintain optimal muscle tissue and metabolism.

What affects Basal Metabolic Rate?

1. Muscle Mass
2. Exercise
3. Meal frequency
4. Meal portion sizes
5. Internal organ function (e.g. enzyme production, liver function, digestion, waste excretion)
6. Body fat levels
7. Genetics
8. Hormonal stress
9. Thermogensis (is the process of heat production)
10. Age

Interesting fact: to gain half a kilo of fat, 3500 calories must be consumed above calories burned which includes basal metabolic rate. Most extreme weight gain found in people may be explained by being water weight. This can also be caused from not consuming enough calories and or yo – yo eating causing severe starvation and hormonal responses.

Chapter Seventeen

THE DANGERS OF YO – YO AND EXTREME DIETING

Dieting (restricting calories) can and will cause loss of lean muscle tissue and will cause the endocrine system to excrete enzymes to help preserve fat to preserve life. Dieting is classed as any food type that restricts calories below basal metabolic rate. This is not safe, can cause death and will cause your body to adapt into a starvation state. Starvation can be classified into five stages, as seen in the table below:

	The 5 Stages of Starvation	
Stage 1	0-8 hours	Absorbs fuel from previous meals
Stage 2	8-10 hours	50% of energy comes from free fatty acids and glycogen storage from the muscles and liver
Stage 3	1-2 days	Body relies on free fatty acids, liver glycogen is completely depleted
Stage 4	After 3 days	Body relies on free fatty acids, increases production of glucose from protein and other fuels. Most tissues are decreasing the use of glucose and body functions start to slow.
Stage 5	After 3-5 days	Metabolic processes slow to preserve energy, protein's via gluconegenesis (a chemical transition of amino acids to glucose) is transposed for energy. This leaving muscle tissue and all other tissue needing protein left without adequate levels therefore causing major muscle loss

The 5 Stages of Starvation		
		and decreased metabolism. After such stress, the endocrine system's preserving enzymes may take up to 2-3 weeks to reduce back to normal levels. Meaning all food brought back into normal daily consumption may be stored; this can cause body fat levels to rise rapidly.

Bio-impedance analysis is an accurate, safe, non invasive means to determine an individual's basal metabolic rate and determine ones state of health and well being. This helps to understand calorie needs for optimal health and fat loss or muscle gain. I have been practicing in bio-impedance testing for years. Visit my website www.threehealthaustralia.com.au for more information.

Chapter Eighteen

THE EASY HAND METHOD

By utilizing the easy hand method, not only will estimating meal portion size be easy but can also be used everywhere you go.

It is a very easy way to approximate the right serving of each macro-nutrient **Carbohydrates, protein and fats**.

I classify **Carbohydrates** as either favorable or non-favorable.

Favorable being **two FIST** size portions like vegetables and salads.

Non-favorable being **one FIST** size portions of potatoes, rice, pasta, cereals and high glycemic carbohydrates like fruit.

Your **Protein** portion should be equal to the size and thickness of your **PALM**.

Use your **THUMB** as an easy measure of the good **Fats**.

The real secret is balancing every meal you eat, every day, every time.

62   *Secrets to a Flatter Stomach*

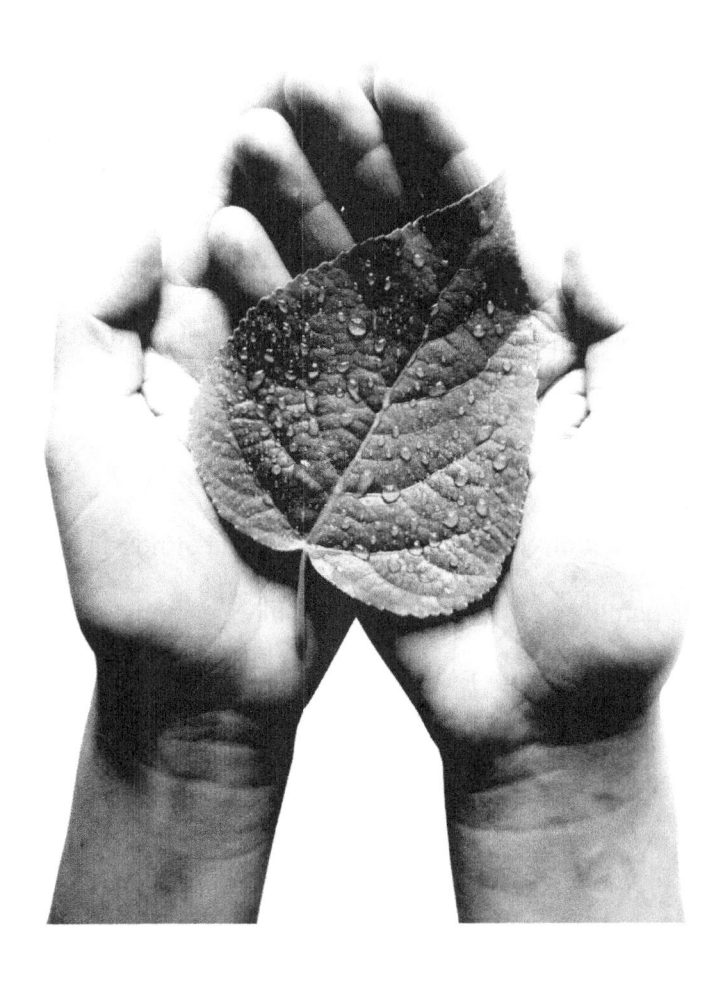

Chapter Nineteen

SPECIFIC NUTRITION PLANNING FOR IDEAL RECOVERY

Here is a sample nutrition plan for a basal metabolic rate of 2280 calories per day when targeting fat loss.
DIVIDE BY NUMBER OF MEALS PER DAY = 4 – 6

EXAMPLE = PER 5 MEALS PER DAY

40 % CARBS = 182 calories ÷ 4 grams = 46 grams
30 % PROTEIN = 136 calories ÷ 4 grams = 34 grams
30 % FATS = 136 calories ÷ 9 grams = 15 grams

Nutrition has its biggest impact during the first 45 minutes post exercise or as we like to call it 'the metabolic window'. To take advantage of this window is to optimize exercise recovery and training adaptation. The muscle cells potential to initiate rebuilding and replenishment peaks about 15 minutes after exercise and declines by as much as 40% within 60 minutes. This window has a major effect of the muscle cells anabolic process, including glycogen storage and protein synthesis. Your post exercise training meal would consist mainly of high glycemic carbohydrates, whey protein and vitamins in liquid form.

I suggest 48 – 80 grams **High Glycemic Carbohydrates** like organic rice milk, glucose, sucrose or maltodextrin
Whey Protein Isolate and/or Concentrate Combination 12 – 40 grams
Creatine 5 – 10 grams
L-Glutamine 5 - 10 grams
Cacao Beans – 8-10
Goji Berries – 1-2 Tablespoons
Zinc/Magnesium Combination – 2-3 capsules

Post (after) Exercise Meal Requirements For This Metabolic Rate

We restrict healthy fats post exercise to create a higher insulin spike for a faster delivery into the cells to provide the greatest recovery.

Carbohydrates = 80 grams   Protein = 34 grams

Chapter Twenty

WHAT TO EAT

Poor nutrition can have a huge impact on your health, well-being, happiness, mood, energy, and focus just to name a few. Conditions like obesity and metabolic syndrome, and such common diseases as cardiovascular disease, diabetes, and osteoporosis. In general, eating a wide variety of fresh, whole (unprocessed) foods have proven favorable compared to diets based on processed foods. Whole foods are those such as fresh tomatoes picked from the garden and red potatoes versus canned tomatoes and instant potatoes.

In particular, the consumption of whole-plant foods slows digestion and allows better absorption, and a more favorable balance of essential nutrients per calorie, as well as better regulation of appetite and blood sugar. Regularly scheduled meals (every 3-4 hours) have also proven more wholesome and aid with a higher body fat loss due to greater metabolic breakdown and hopefully smaller portions.

There are seven major classes of nutrients:

1. Carbohydrates
2. Fats
3. Protein
4. Fiber
5. Minerals
6. Vitamins
7. Water.

The macronutrients are carbohydrates, fats, fiber, proteins, and water.

The micronutrients are minerals and vitamins. Vitamins, minerals, fiber, and water do not provide energy, but are necessary for all other chemical functions in your body. Think of micronutrients as the breakdown of the whole macronutrients we eat. Micronutrients are nutrients required by the body for a huge range of physiological and chemical functions. Most foods contain a mix of some or all of the nutrient classes. Some nutrients are required regularly, while others are needed only occasionally. Poor health can be caused by an imbalance of nutrients, whether an excess or a deficiency.

Some examples of minerals are iron, cobalt, copper, sulfur, iodine, manganese, selenium, chromium and molybdenum. Some examples of vitamins are vitamin A, vitamin B (B1, B2, B3, B5, B6, B7 and B12), vitamin C, vitamin D, vitamin E, and vitamin K. Vitamins are classified as either water-soluble or fat soluble. There are 13 vitamins: 4 fat-soluble (A, D, E and K) and 9 water-soluble (B vitamins and vitamin C). Water-soluble vitamins dissolve easily in water, and in general, are easily excreted from the body. Because they are not readily stored, consistent daily intake is important.

Fat-soluble vitamins are absorbed through the intestinal tract with the help of fats. Because they are more likely to accumulate in the body, in general we don't need to consume as much or as often.

In general the micronutrient quality depends solely from the quality of soil and farming techniques. Micronutrient deficiencies are worldwide. Approximately 50% of world cereal soils are deficient in zinc and 30% of cultivated soils are deficient in iron. Organic crops host a higher quality of these micronutrients compared to non-organic crops.

Using the ratio of 40% Carbohydrates, 30% Protein and 30% Fat and selecting a variety of colour food types will help maintain optimal weight, optimal hormonal levels, general weight and good health.

PROTEIN		
Favorable choice	Fair choice	Poor choice
Chicken breast, deli style	Cheese, reduced fat	Hard cheeses
Chicken breast, skinless	Mozzarella cheese, skim	Bacon
Turkey breast, deli style	Ricotta cheese, skim	Beef, fatty cuts
Turkey breast, skinless	Beef, lean cuts	Beef; ground (more
Bass	Bacon, lean	than 10% fat)
Bluefish	Chicken, dark meat, lean	Hot dog (turkey or
Calamari	Duck	chicken)
Catfish	Ham, deli style	Liver, beef
Cod	Ham, lean	Liver, chicken
Clams	Lamb, lean	Pepperoni
Crabmeat	Pork, lean	Pork sausage

PROTEIN		
Favorable choice	Fair choice	Poor choice
Haddock
Halibut
Lobster
Mackerel
Salmon
Sardines
Scallops
Snapper
Swordfish
Trout
Tuna (steak)
Tuna, canned in water
Prawns
Protein powder
Soy burgers
Soy hot dog
Soy sausages
Tofu, firm or extra firm
Egg whites
Cheese fat free
Cottage cheese, low fat
Cottage cheese, no fat
Milk, low fat 1%
Tempeh
Yoghurt, plain	Pork chop
Turkey, dark meat, skinless
Turkey bacon
Veal	Salami

CARBOHYDRATES		
Favorable choice	Fair choice	Poor choice
Artichoke
Asparagus
Beans, black canned
Beans, green or wax
Bok Choy
Broccoli
Brussels sprouts
Cabbage	Acorn squash
Baked beans
Beetroot
Carrots
Corn
Lima beans
Parsnips
Peas	Barbeque sauce
Sugar bar's
Cocktail sauce
Graham cracker
Saltine crackers
Honey
Premium ice cream
Regular ice cream

CARBOHYDRATES		
Favorable choice	Fair choice	Poor choice
Cauliflower Chickpeas Collard greens Eggplant Kale Kidney beans Leeks Lentils Mushrooms Okra Onions boiled Sauerkraut Spinach Swiss chard Turnip Turnip, greens Yellow squash Zucchini **Raw vegetables** Alfalfa Bean sprouts Broccoli Cabbage Cauliflower Celery Cucumber Endive Escarole Green capsicumGreen capsicum Hummus Lettuce, ice berg Lettuce romaine Mushrooms Onions Radishes Salsa Snow peas Spinach	Pinto beans Potato, baked Potato, boiled Potato French fried Potato mashed Pumpkin Refried beans Sweet potato baked Sweet potato mashed **Fruit** Cranberries Cranberry sauce Dates Fig Guava Kumquat Mango Papaya Prunes Raisins **Fruit juices** Apple cider Apple juice Cranberry juice Fruit punch Grape juice Grapefruit juice Lemon juice Lemonade Orange juice Pineapple juice Tomato juice V-8 juice **Grains cereals and breads** Bagel small Biscuit	Jam or jelly Molasses Plum sauce Potato chips Pretzels Relish, pickle Brown sugar Confectioners' sugar Granulated sugar Maple syrup Pancake syrup Tomato sauce Teriyaki sauce Tortilla chips

CARBOHYDRATES		
Favorable choice	Fair choice	Poor choice
Spinach salad Tomatoes **Fruit: fresh, frozen or canned light** Apple Applesauce Apricots Blackberries Blueberries Cantaloupe Cherries Fruit cocktail Grapefruit Grapes Honeydew melon Kiwi Lemon Lime Nectarine Orange Mandarin Peach Peaches Pear Pineapple Plum Raspberries Strawberries Tangerine Watermelon Grains Oats	Bread wholegrain Bread white Bread crumbs Breadstick Buckwheat dry Bulgur wheat dry Cereal dry Cornbread Cornstarch Couscous Croissant plain Crouton Donut plain English muffin Granola Melba toast Millet Muffin Egg noodles 4 inch pancake Cooked pasta Pita bread Mini pita bread Popcorn Brown rice White rice Roll, dinner Hamburger roll Taco shell Corn tortilla Flour tortilla Waffle	

FATS		
Favorable choice	Fair choice	Poor choice
Almond butter Almonds	Mayonnaise light Mayonnaise regular	Bacon bits imitation Butter

FATS		
Favorable choice	Fair choice	Poor choice
Avocado Slivered almonds Canola oil Flaxseeds Guacamole Linseeds Macadamia nuts Olive oil Olive oil & vinegar dressing Olives Peanut butter, natural Peanut oil Peanuts Tahini Sunflower seeds	Sesame oil Soybean oil Walnuts	Cream Cream cheese Light cream cheese Lard Sour cream Sour cream light Vegetable shortening

Part 3

Detoxification

"our ultimate form of natural protection."

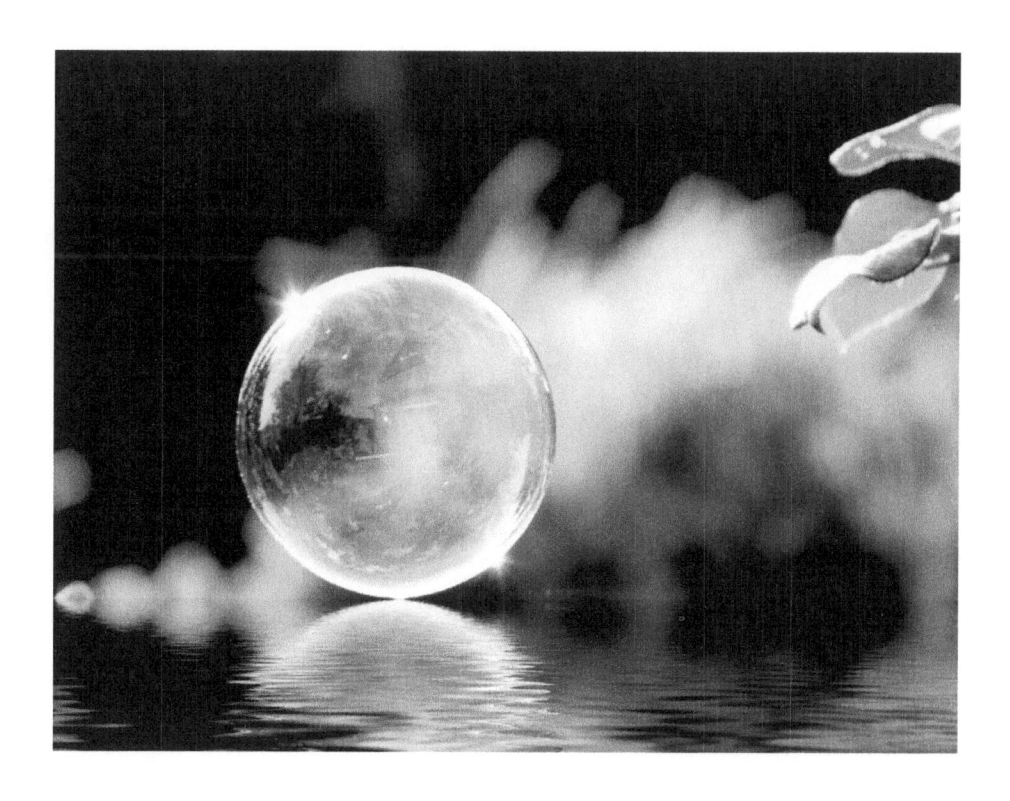

Chapter Twenty-one

TOXINS

Toxins are impurities that damage our body in different ways. Unfortunately even the most health concerned individual finds it extremely hard to be toxin free. Toxins are everywhere. We come into contact with three type of toxins everyday:

1. Toxins we absorb externally through the skin and nose.
2. Toxins we ingest when we eat.
3. Toxins or free radicals we produce from exercise or when we become stressed.

Our bodies can easily become 'toxic' when our cleansing systems become clogged, sluggish and overloaded or stressed.

Toxins are either fat soluble or water soluble. Water soluble toxins are eliminated via excretion. Fat soluble toxins are stored in fat cells. Fat soluble toxins make utilizing and burning energy from particular areas of our body's fat harder. This may explain some contribution to problematic areas. The skin will absorb both water and fat soluble toxins depositing them straight into the blood stream. Stress, an excess of body's natural chemicals and cumulative life experiences also promotes toxic build up within the body and enhances hormone imbalances. In addition to these, toxic overload may contribute to more serious conditions such as autoimmune diseases including inflammatory and rheumatoid arthritis and neurological diseases such as Alzheimer's and Parkinson's disease.

To add to problems, toxic overload can manifest in a number of ways, this may include, headaches, muscle and joint pain, mental confusion (often linked with candida), gastrointestinal tract irregularities, slow cellular metabolism, fatigue, depression, clogged skin, flu like symptoms, poor body fat break down and even allergic reactions. Susceptibility and response to toxins varies with age, gender, genetic factors, nutritional habits and lifestyle. Today's children are at the highest risk because of modern food changes, fast food choices and chemicals/preservatives introduced into foods.

When researches first discovered nutrients that help cleanse the body, they were looking for ways to prevent deadly diseases caused by toxic burden. Dr Bruce N Ames PhD, professor of molecular and cell biology at the University of California notes; the body has 7 channels for detoxification and elimination, with the increasing demand for more food and the use of more and more chemicals, he believes cleanses will provide specific support to eliminate the overload of toxins that we are exposed to and ingest.

The seven channels for human detoxification are as follows

The bowels, blood, skin, kidneys, lymphatic system, lungs and the most important being the liver. He states 'they all work individually and as a team'. If any one of these channels of elimination is not functioning well, health declines. The liver is the largest gland and is the main chemical processing plant for the body. It processes all foreign waste and eliminates toxic wastes. The cleaner your liver, the leaner you will be.

The liver is also a primary player in your body's immune system. An overburdened liver only disposes of small amounts of impurities whilst other toxins are stored in the liver's cells, eventually causing irreversible damage. The liver has many functions; the main function is elimination of toxins. It also metabolizes fats, protein and carbohydrates, breaks down and eliminates hormones, stores vitamins, minerals and sugars. Pharmaceuticals, even though ingested for medical purposes, are synthetic and cause extreme stress on the liver. Supporting your liver, limiting your exposure to toxins, undertaking liver flushes and herbal treatments, increasing your amount of healthy fluids and limiting late night activities (this is when the liver under goes rebuilding) can be big steps in supporting healthy immunity and optimum liver function.

Detoxification is extremely important in your quest for the optimal looking and optimal functioning body. This may answer questions why some people have no trouble losing weight and why some people keep adding weight. It is not uncommon for someone to add 1/2 Kg of toxic weight in one year. I believe that detoxification is the missing link, it can be more important to someone than any exercise and nutritional prescribed program.

Unfortunately detoxification has a bad reputation. Most likely caused by poor administration, lack of knowledge and the severe extremity of the program. Most people may also look for the easy fix, unfortunately toxins have taken some, if not, a lifetime to congest and build up in your system. In desperation or in the belief from uneducated professionals, may promise toxic build up to be flushed out in only a matter of weeks and in some cases, days. This is simply not the case. The good news is that if you've suffered the negative impact of an overly toxic/acidic body, you can regain your health.

Advantages of Detoxification

Detoxification administered properly and using simple old fashioned techniques make it easier to:

- ✓ Manage weight
- ✓ Increased basal metabolic rate
- ✓ Increases energy levels
- ✓ Supports healthy immunity
- ✓ Helps manage appetite
- ✓ Curbs sugar cravings
- ✓ Maintains colon health and regularity
- ✓ Helps maintain healthy cholesterol and triglycerides
- ✓ Helps improve absorption of vitamins and minerals
- ✓ Helps normalize blood pressure
- ✓ Maximizes fat utilization when exercising

Because of the impact some detoxification programs have on the elimination of medical supplements, eliminating their effectiveness, a supplement program for detoxification is out of the scope of this book and I would recommend you seek professional advice when deciding to detoxify your system. Whilst many so called exercise experts may promote a 'no need to detoxify', I'm a realist and believe the total amount of chemicals and cheap ways to produce food over burdens our systems. Even though the most motivated individual may need and try to consume up to 1.5 kilograms of green vegetables and purchase and drink at least 4-6 litres or pure water per day may struggle to continue the trend needed to cleanse naturally. The key to regaining health is consuming alkaline foods and liquids. They aid in absorbing and excreting toxins within our system.

Interesting fact: Why are diet soft drinks so bad? How could it possibly make me gain weight, it's zero calories? Diet soft drinks and normal soft drinks contain artificial sweeteners which are 100% chemicals which need purification. This forces our bodies into an acidic state. Our bodies are constantly putting mechanisms in place to keep our blood pH neutral. Every food and drink is alkaline, acidic or neutral. These levels are measured in pH (potential of hydrogen). These range from 0-14 pH. 0 being the most acidic, 14 the most alkaline and 7 classed as neutral.

Some common pH examples include: stomach acid equaling 1, diet soft drinks 2.5, coffee 3, water at 7 and our blood is at 7.35. Our body will not allow our pH to become imbalanced because if it did we would become toxic and die. Our body increase respiration, perspiration, urination and will use important minerals to reach balance when we ingest acidic food or drinks. Diet and normal soft drink causes our body to use important alkalising minerals like calcium, magnesium, iodine, potassium and sodium to compensate and return pH to normal. Diet soft drinks and normal soft drinks contain phosphoric acid (also used in "rust remover" or "rust killer" solutions for cleaning metals) and often other chemical sweeteners. For example: Iodine helps support the thyroid gland, without iodine the thyroid cannot function efficiently. The thyroid gland controls metabolic rate. Lack of iodine causes an inefficient thyroid gland causing an increase in weight gain and poor functioning thyroid! Diet Soft drinks steal iodine to help balance pH therefore leaving the thyroid to function inefficiently.

Alkalizing and Acidifying Foods

The following list provides information about the various food substances to whether they provide acidifying or alkalizing reactions provided by 'The Wolfe Clinic'. The presence of high acidity indicates more of your foods should be selected from the alkalizing group. In general, it is important to have a diet that contains foods from both groups, but including more from the alkaline groupings. Alkaline foods also play a major factor in reducing toxins and free radicals in your body. For the most, it will be nearly impossible to select only alkaline types and I recommend you don't try to. As you see in the list below most protein sources are acidic. If you try to consume 100% of your foods from alkaline types you risk the chance of loss of muscle tissue which can cause a slower basal metabolic rate. A ratio of 60%

Alkaline:40% Acidic has been shown to be extremely effective in overall health and fat loss.

	ALKALISING FOODS
Vegetables	Garlic, Asparagus, Fermented Veggies, Watercress, Beets, Broccoli, Brussel sprouts, Cabbage, Carrot, Cauliflower, Celery, Chard, Chlorella, Collard Greens, Cucumber, Eggplant, Kale, Kohlrabi, Lettuce, Mushrooms, Mustard Greens, Dulce, Dandelions, Edible Flowers, Onions, Parsnips (high glycemic), Peas, Peppers, Pumpkin, Rutabaga, Sea Veggies, Spirulina, Sprouts, Squashes, Alfalfa, Barley Grass, Wheat Grass, Wild Greens, Nightshade Veggies.
Fruits	Apple, Apricot, Avocado, Banana (high glycemic), Cantaloupe, Cherries, Currants, Dates/Figs, Grapes, Grapefruit, Lime, Honeydew Melon, Nectarine, Orange, Lemon Peach, Pear, Pineapple, All Berries, Tangerine, Tomato, Tropical Fruits, Watermelon
Protein	Free range eggs, whey protein powder, fat free cottage cheese, organic yogurt, almonds, chestnuts, tofu, flaxseeds, pumpkin seeds, tempeh, squash seeds, sunflower seeds, millet, and nuts.
Beverages	Vegetable juices, fresh fruit juice, organic milk, mineral water, quality water above 7.45ph, Stevia (natural sweetner)
Teas	Green tea, herbal, dandelion, ginseng, bancha, kombucha.
Spices and Seasonings	Cinnamon, curry, ginger, mustard, chili peppers, salt (sea salt), miso, tamari, all herbs

ACIDIFYING FOODS	
Fats and Oils	Avocado oil, canola oil, corn oil, hemp seed oil, flax oil, grape seed oil, lard, olive oil, safflower oil, sesame oil, sunflower oil.
Fruits	Cranberries
Grains	Rice cakes, wheat cakes, barley, buckwheat, corn, oats, rice (brown, basmati), rye, spelt, kamut, wheat, hemp seed flour.
Dairy, Milke and Hard Cheese	Cow cheese, goat cheese, processed cheese, sheep cheese, milk.
Nuts and Butter	Cashews, filberts, Brazil nuts, peanuts, peanut butter, butters, pecans, Tahini, walnuts.
Animal Protein	Rabbit, salmon, prawns, scallops, tuna, turkey, venison, Lean chicken breast, beef, carp, clams, duck, fish, white meat, lamb, lobster, mussels, oyster, pork,
Pasta	Noodles, macaroni, spaghetti.
Others	Distilled vinegar, brewer's yeast, wheat germ, potatoes
Drugs and Chemicals	All chemicals and medicines, pesticides, herbicides.
Sweets and Sweetners	Molasses, candy, chocolate, honey, maple syrup, saccharin, sucrolose, soft drinks, sugars, aspartame, fruit flavored drinks, any diet products.
Alcholic Beverages	Beers, spirits, hard liquor, wine
Beans and Legumes	Black beans, chick beans, green peas, kidney beans, lentils, lima beans, pinto beans, red beans, soybeans, soy milk, white beans.

Chapter Twenty-two

ANTI-OXIDANTS AND FREE RADICALS

Anti-oxidants repair and prevent damage to all our living cells. Every cell in the body needs oxygen to carry on its individual functions; oxygen is however, a reactive substance and reacts with other substances, this cause's oxidation. Anti-oxidants' main properties are not cleansing; they are repairing and preventing further damage to all our living cells. Free radicals are destructive chemicals produced naturally during metabolism that cause damage of cell membranes and DNA and promotes heart disease, cancer, high cholesterol and pre-mature ageing. Researchers have determined that this oxidation causes cells to die and is one of the primary causes of pre- mature ageing.

The biochemical forms of oxygen that are most likely to cause pre-mature ageing are commonly known as 'Free Radicals'. Free radicals are molecules that are missing an electron, so they steal a replacement electron from another molecule, causing oxidative damage to the victimized molecule and the tissue of which it is a part of. Unfortunately, free radicals cause a huge domino effect in the body and we are constantly battling to get enough nutrients from foods to avoid damage. Anti-oxidants are our first line of defense against free radical damage. The ORAC Level is the rating of free radical absorption by a type of food or liquid.

Here is a list showing the highest ORAC levels per 100 grams:

1. Raw Cacao Beans – 95,500
2. Goji Berries – 25,300
3. Acai Berries – 18,500
4. Dark Chocolate 70% Cacao or higher – 13,120
5. Prunes – 5770
6. Pomegranates - 3307

7. Raisins – 2830
8. Blueberries – 2400
9. Blackberries – 2036
10. Garlic - 1939
11. Kale – 1770
12. Spinach – 1260

Oil Types:
1. Clove Oil – 10,786,875
2. Thyme Oil – 159,590
3. Oregano Oil – 153,007

Food supplements also can be effective

Here is a list of anti-oxidant supplements that have been thoroughly researched and that I recommend. Please seek the advice of a healthcare professional before taking any new supplements.

- **Alpha Lipoic Acid** -Universal anti-oxidant because of its ability to work on both water and fat soluble toxins and has evidence that it protects against cancer and been successfully used to treat diabetes and hepatitis C.
- **CO Enzyme Q10** - Fat soluble, regenerates Vitamin E in the anti-oxidant network. Used for heart disease, rejuvenates brain cells and helps prevent Alzheimer's and Parkinson's disease. A must if you have high cholesterol or taking lower agents.
- **L-Glutathione** - Scavenges free radicals in the brain and protects against radiation, pesticides, chemicals and heavy metals. Enhances Vitamin A and E. Inhibits certain enzymes that break down collagen in the skin. This also prevents histamine production thereby reducing severity of allergies.
- **Acetyl L-Carnitine** - Helps to body's ability to burn fat as energy.
- **Vitamin C** - Magic immune builder and powerful anti-oxidant.
- **Vitamin E** - Vitamin E is a fat-soluble antioxidant and it helps protects cell membranes from oxidation.

- **Vitamin A** - Vitamin A is a fat-soluble antioxidant which plays a role in a variety of functions throughout the body, such as vision, gene transcription, immune function, embryonic development and skin health.

- **Selenium** - Selenium is a micro nutrient mineral, vital for protective enzymes and also plays a role in the functioning of the thyroid gland.

Chapter Twenty-three

THE IMPORTANCE OF CIRCULATION

Blood is the body's main internal transport system and proper circulation is vital for good health. Circulatory disorders are quite common in middle-ages and elderly people. Hypertension and poor circulation are the most well known. It can be caused by cholesterol plaque deposits along the inner walls of the arteries; the blood then exerts great force against the walls of the blood vessels causing the blood pressure to rise.

Too much body fat, excess water or fluid retention can also cause these problems. Circulatory problems are very prevalent in this age of bad foods, little if any exercise and high stress levels from lifestyle. Circulation from exercise increases blood flow and delivers oxygen to all living cells, without this blood flow, the body's cells start breaking down and premature ageing can take place.

Skin Brushing

If it is impossible for you to exercise then skin brushing your skin each day has been proven to increase blood flow by up to 200%. This will help cleanse your body inside and out, help relieve swollen areas, improve digestion and improve energy levels.

Perform a good skin brushing once or twice a day, especially before showering, bathing, or exercise. A complete skin brushing should take no longer than 2 to 5 minutes. A skin brush is usually made from either horse hair or cactus. Please don't purchase plastic skin brushes as this can also clog your pores even more. Skin brushes can be found at any good health and skin shop. Now, using the brush (dry), stroke your skin (also dry) in long, sweeping strokes. Bear down to achieve a stimulating effect. Pass over every part of your body except for your face and the front of your neck. Do not brush back and forth or in a circular motion. Do not scrub or massage. Always brushing the skin towards the heart. For areas of cellulite, extra stimulation assists the body's ability to decongest.

Skin brushing is highly effective for

- Achieving beautiful radiant skin
- Supporting new cell formation
- Moving congested fluids and edema (water build up)
- Stimulating blood circulation
- Correcting inflammation of the lymph nodes
- Improving body tone

Once the colon is partially cleansed, it takes a few months of skin brushing to completely cleanse the lymphatic system. When practiced daily for several months, five minutes per day is easily worth 30 minutes of vigorous exercise in blood circulation.

Chapter Twenty-four

WHAT ABOUT CHOLESTEROL?

Approx 80% of the cholesterol in our body is produced by your liver; it is a waxy fat like substance. Cholesterol forms part of every cell and serves many vital functions. The remaining comes from our diet. Good Cholesterol or HDL (High density lipoprotein) removes bad cholesterol from within the arteries and transports them back to the liver for excretion. Bad Cholesterol or LDL (Low density lipoprotein) transports cholesterol into the artery wall, which can then attract white blood cells that can easily start the formation of plaques. Over time can cause ruptures, activate blood clotting which if severe can result in heart attack, stroke and cardiovascular disease.

The body makes much of its cholesterol out of saturated fatty acids in foods we eat, such as red meat and butter. It is also created in our body from the breakdown of sugar. Therefore, if your diet consists of high amounts of refined sugar, starch (which becomes sugar), and carbohydrate-rich food (such as white bread), your body will contain a lot of saturated fats and, logically, more cholesterol. You've heard of trans fatty acids, right? Well, eating trans fatty acids raises your levels of bad cholesterol and lowers levels of good cholesterol. Tran's fatty acids are found in most vegetable oils and margarines. Having too much cholesterol in the blood stream can be thought of like honey in your fuel tank. This slows blood circulation causing your heart to pump harder and more frequent, this aiding to higher stress to the heart. Bad cholesterol may also become clogged or attached to the wall linings all throughout our circulatory system. This can easily cause blockage and limit blood supply to vital areas. Cholesterol has many vital functions in our body. Our body needs cholesterol for maintaining healthy walls, hormone production, making vitamin D and producing bile acids which help digestion of fat. These also include healthy brain function, DNA reproduction and general well being.

The reasons why you may have high cholesterol
1. Poor nutrition
2. Too much refined carbohydrate
3. Consuming too many Tran's fatty acids
4. Lack of fiber
5. Genetics
6. Hypothyroidism
7. Stress
8. Lack of exercise
9. Smoking.

Tips you must follow in order to lower cholesterol without using medical lower agents.

- ✓ **Eat less Refined carbohydrates**
- ✓ **Eat more Fiber** (Wheat, rye, oats, barley, legumes and most fruits and vegetables)
- ✓ **Eat the right fats and avoid the bad ones** (Omega 3 fatty acids, flaxseed oil etc)
- ✓ **Increase the Anti-oxidants in your daily nutrition** (Consume an anti-oxidant blend or use super foods)
- ✓ **Ingest herbs to help your heart** (Green tea, garlic, ginger, turmeric)
- ✓ **Improve your liver function** (Milk thistle, taurine, artichokes, schizandra and dandelion root)
- ✓ **Strengthen your immune system** (Avoid foods causing allergies or intolerance, eat raw vegetables, detoxify your body, and take specific vitamins and minerals)
- ✓ **Manage stress levels** (Magnesium, relaxation, sleep, massage, keeps cortisol levels down (zinc, magnesium & B6/B12 combination)
- ✓ **You must exercise** (2 to 5 days per week for 20 – 60 minutes.

Conclusion

IT'S UP TO YOU

Self discipline is defined in many ways.

adopt a particular pattern of behavior even though one would rather be doing something else'

'is the commitment to a goal, the ability to maintain a dedicated amount of time and effort to a task until the goal is reached'

'is having the will power, self control and self motivation to achieve what you desire to achieve, confronting the brutal facts and not letting excuses take control'

'having a mental and physical ability to go through with set tasks regardless of whether you want to or not'

'controlling one's behavior either by self or by a third party acting sensibly and responsibly even when instincts and emotion might be itching you to act opposing'

'is being able to abide by a set of standards and rules over a period of time'

What would you think if I said you're success relies solely on your own ability to be self disciplined? I have heard numerous times from people, clients, know it all's, 'oh I tried that program and it did nothing'! Let me share with you the reality.

After recently having a work colleague stay with me, I have witnessed first hand how well my health and fitness program works! Or as we see, how well it doesn't!

Let's go back 2 months. My good friend and work colleague asked me for help. 'Whatever it takes' he tells me, I promise to do whatever you think I need to do. I set up a 12 week program, mapping out everything he needs to do, exercise programming, nutrition design and even set him up a simple yet effective detoxification program to help reduce his high cholesterol and to help speed up fat loss. Approximately 4 week in, he explained he felt he had hit a plateau, no longer getting the results he wanted. After consulting his nutrition, exercise program, he honestly told me he was doing everything I asked him to do. 2 weeks ago he needed a place to stay and obviously I offered without second thought. I sneakily watched his daily patterns. The results were interesting to say the least.

In the first week, he missed breakfast 4 out of the 7 days and consumed Chinese takeaway 3 times for dinner, 'Yeah been a busy week, I thought Chinese was a healthy choice?' . He completed 1 of the 3 early morning walks and completed 2 out of the 3 strength training sessions. So far he has followed my program approximately 40%. The second week didn't get much better. Although he did do all the morning walks and completed 2 out of the 3 strength sessions, breakfast was again seriously overlooked.

The takeaway foods for dinner were still consumed 3 times and to top things off, whilst taking the rubbish out, I noticed a whole stack of empty full strength beer cans.

So a plateau? My program abused with little results. So the program is definitely at fault!

No doubt the same with the millions of program's available in which people have attempted. Don't get me wrong, there are some seriously downright bad high risk exercise programs with unattainable meal plans handed out every single day. But, I'm sure self-discipline is the reasoning behind most failures.

What contributes you from getting mediocre results to amazing results?

Your success truly relies on your own self discipline. You now have all the tools to succeed, to become educated, to become fit, healthy and regain your life or take your physique above and beyond.

Ask yourself…

What I am willing to do in order to succeed?

What am I willing to let go of in order to achieve?

Nine Steps to Self-Discipline

1. For disciplined actions first needs disciplined thoughts
2. Commit yourself completely
3. Be realistic and brutally honest with yourself

4. Be accountable and don't make excuses
5. Follow the plan and prepare each day
6. Discipline yourself from temptation
7. Write down everything you do and re-read every second day
8. Maintain a positive outlook and never give up
9. Believe in yourself and enjoy your success

'The difference between a successful person and others is not a lack of strength nor knowledge but rather is a lack of will and desire'

Vince Lombardi

Summary

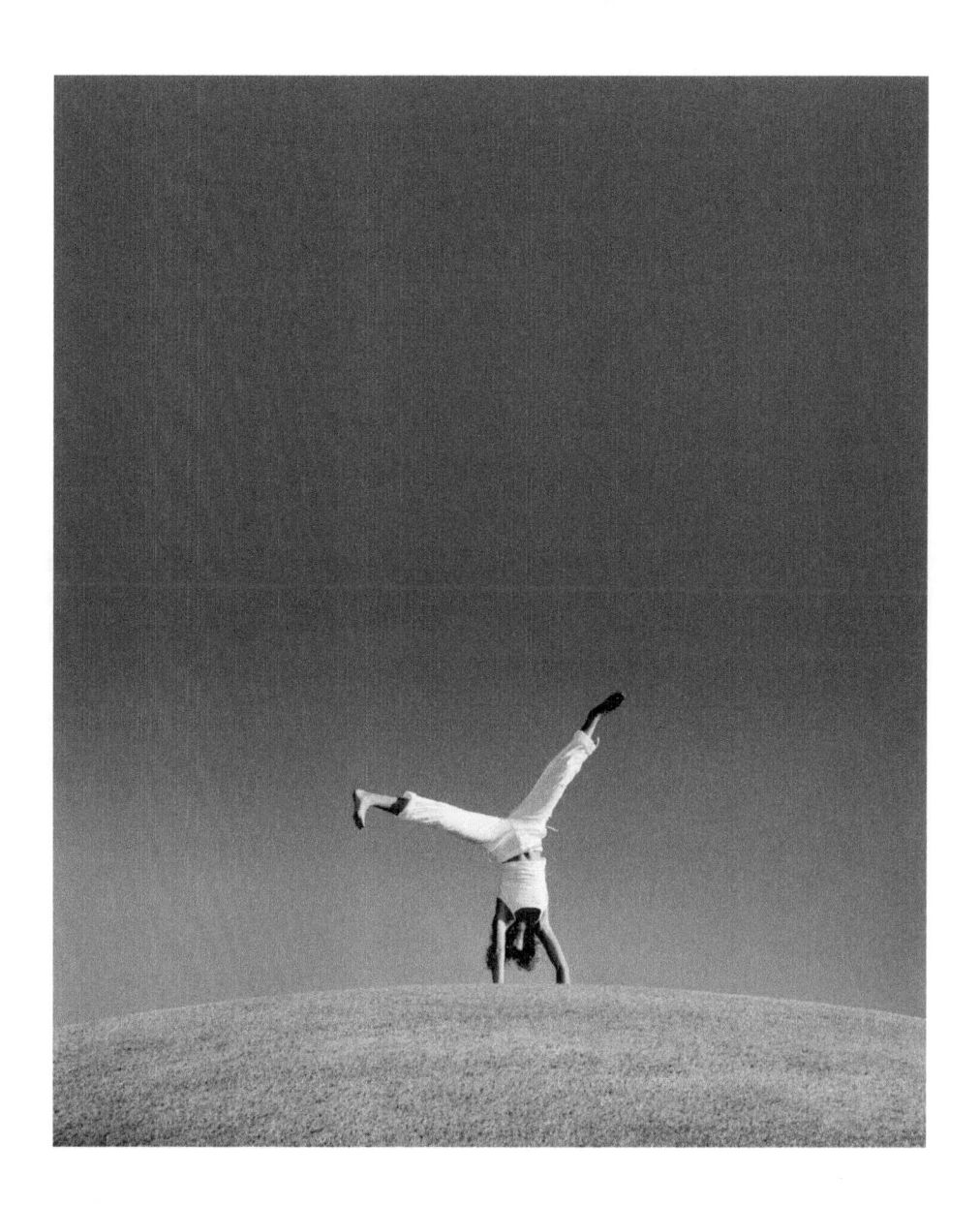

Here are the main points I want you to remember:

1. Exercise makes up approximately 30-40% of your result, so relax and enjoy your exercise.
2. Strength training is a must for everyone, complete your strength training first followed by your cardiovascular training to maximize fat burning.
3. Train smart and use scientific programming.
4. Exercise consistently - changing your program every 4-6 weeks.
5. Balance your meals using the hand method to approximate portion control as much as possible.
6. Make sure you consume enough balanced calories equaling (at minimum) your basal metabolic rate divided every 3-4 hours.
7. Eat real food, lean protein and as much dark green vegetables as possible.
8. Be realistic and follow a scientific nutrition plan.
9. If your number one goal is fat loss, you must exercise in a carbohydrate depleted state, complete 30-45 minutes cardiovascular exercise before breakfast.
10. If your number one goal is muscle gain, you must consume enough calories, consume a medium GI carbohydrate meal 45 minutes before strength training and consume a high GI carbohydrate and protein meal within 30-45 minutes post exercise.
11. Participate in a detoxification program, depending on your current state of health will depend on how long you need to detoxify for. Please seek professional advice before starting any detoxification program.
12. Make sleep a priority. Stress kills, relax and enjoy your life.
13. If you are not seeing results, make a change.
14. Continue to educate yourself. Reading more health and fitness books will help keep you motivated and keep you up to date with all the latest research.

You are an unrepeatable miracle. Never Give Up. You are worth it.

'Do today what others won't so you can live tomorrow like others can't.'

Unknown

My favourite statement – Eat well, train hard and rest more!

Yours in health and fitness,
Time to shine….

Jamie Flynn
THREE HEALTH AUSTRALIA
www.threehealthaustralia.com.au

References and Acknowledgements

Secrets to a Flatter Stomach was created and written by Jamie Flynn based on his successful educational seminar. Edited and published by Lulu.com

Qualifications - Cert III and IV Level 1 Master Trainer (Australian Institute Of Fitness) Les Mills Personal Trainer (Nutrition) - Steiner UK London Accredited (Mat Yoga, Pilates & Freestyle Indoor Cycling) - Les Mills Accredited (Boxing & Kickboxing for fun and fitness) - Accredited Fit Ball Australia - St John's Senior First Aid.

Experience - 12 years Personal Training - Senior Lecturer & Course Coach (Australian Institute of Fitness) - Weight loss & Strength Training Coach - Natural Body Building Specialist - Metabolic Analysis Specialist (BIA System - Polar Body Age System) - TRX Suspension Trainer - Detoxification & Specific Nutrition Specialist - Lifestyle Coach & Motivational Speaker.

References

- Fitness Leaders Handbook: A lot of early knowledge came from this book. Published book – Authored by Larry Egger and Nigel Champion.
- United States Department of Agriculture: The USDA website can be cited at www.usda.gov
- American College of Sports Medicine: Website information can be found at www.acsm.org
- American Heart Association: www.americanheart.org
- Australian Heart Association: www.heartfoundation.org.au
- Australian Institute of Fitness – Perth, Australia: Much of my general knowledge came from the certification I received from their course. www.fitness.edu.au

- The Wolfe Clinic: www.thewolfeclinic.com
- How to eat, move and be healthy: Published book – Authored by Paul Chek
- Beyond Brawn: Published book – Authored by Stuart McRobert
- Look good, feel great: Published book – Authored by Stephen J Smith
- The Zone Diet : Published book – Authored by Dr Barry Sears
- The Performance Zone: Published book – Authored by Dr John Ivy and Dr Robert Portman
- Cholesterol-The Real Truth: Published book – Authored by Dr Sandra Cabot
- The Ketogenic Diet: Published book – Authored by Lyle McDonald
- Anabolic Diet: Published book – Dr Mauro Di Pasquale
- Modern Nutrition in Health and Disease: Published book – Maurice Edward Shils
- Wiki – Wikipedia: The free encyclopedia www.en.wikipedia.org
- Personal Trainers: Shawn Baxter, James Miller, Martin Toomey, Wayne Zimmer